Controversies in Equine Medicine and Surgery

Editor

ROBERT J. MacKAY

VETERINARY CLINICS
OF NORTH AMERICA:
EQUINE PRACTICE

www.vetequine.theclinics.com

Consulting Editor
THOMAS J. DIVERS

August 2019 • Volume 35 • Number 2

ELSEVIER

1600 John F. Kennedy Boulevard • Suite 1800 • Philadelphia, Pennsylvania, 19103-2899

http://www.vetequine.theclinics.com

VETERINARY CLINICS OF NORTH AMERICA: EQUINE PRACTICE Volume 35, Number 2
August 2019 ISSN 0749-0739, ISBN-13: 978-0-323-68219-0

Editor: Colleen Dietzler
Developmental Editor: Donald Mumford

Veterinary Clinics of North America: Equine Practice (ISSN 0749-0739) is published in April, August, and December by Elsevier Inc., 360 Park Avenue South, New York, NY 10010-1710. Business and Editorial Offices: 1600 John F. Kennedy Blvd., Suite 1800, Philadelphia, PA 19103-2899. Subscription prices are $287.00 per year (domestic individuals), $557.00 per year (domestic institutions), $100.00 per year (domestic students/residents), $334.00 per year (Canadian individuals), $702.00 per year (Canadian institutions), $365.00 per year (international individuals), $702.00 per year (international institutions), and $180.00 per year (international and Canadian students/residents). To receive student/resident rate, orders must be accompanied by name of affiliated institution, date of term, and the signature of program/residency coordinator on institution letterhead. Orders will be billed at individual rate until proof of status is received. Foreign air speed delivery is included in all *Clinics* subscription prices. All prices are subject to change without notice. **POSTMASTER:** Send address changes to *Veterinary Clinics of North America: Equine Practice*, 3251 Riverport Lane, Maryland Heights, MO 63043. Customer Service (orders, claims, online, change of address): Elsevier Health Sciences Division, Subscription **Customer Service, 3251 Riverport Lane, Maryland Heights, MO 63043. Tel: 1-800-654-2452 (U.S. and Canada); 314-447-8871 (outside U.S. and Canada). Fax: 314-447-8029. E-mail: journalscustomerservice-usa@elsevier.com (for print support);** E-mail: **journalsonlinesupport-usa@elsevier. com (for online support).**

Reprints. For copies of 100 or more of articles in this publication, please contact the Commercial Reprints Department, Elsevier Inc., 360 Park Avenue South, New York, NY 10010-1710. Tel.: 212-633-3874; Fax: 212-633-3820; E-mail: reprints@elsevier.com.

Veterinary Clinics of North America: Equine Practice is covered in *MEDLINE/PubMed (Index Medicus), Excerpta Medica, Current Contents/Agriculture, Biology and Environmental Sciences,* and *ISI.*

Contributors

CONSULTING EDITOR

THOMAS J. DIVERS, DVM
Diplomate, American College of Veterinary Internal Medicine; Diplomate, American College of Veterinary Emergency and Critical Care; Steffen Professor of Veterinary Medicine, Department of Clinical Sciences, Section of Large Animal Medicine, Cornell University College of Veterinary Medicine, Ithaca, New York, USA

EDITOR

ROBERT J. MacKAY, BVSc (Dist), PhD
Diplomate, American College of Veterinary Internal Medicine; Professor, Department of Large Animal Clinical Sciences, University of Florida, Gainesville, Florida, USA

AUTHORS

CHELSIE A. BURDEN, DVM, MS
Diplomate, American College of Theriogenologists; Associate, Goulburn Valley Equine Hospital, Congupna, Victoria, Australia

TERESA A. BURNS, DVM, PhD
Assistant Professor, Department of Veterinary Clinical Studies, College of Veterinary Medicine, The Ohio State University, Columbus, Ohio, USA

ELEANOR J. CRISPE, BVMS, PhD
Senior Veterinarian, Simon Miller Racing, Shenton Park, Western Australia, Australia

THOMAS J. DIVERS, DVM
Diplomate, American College of Veterinary Internal Medicine; Diplomate, American College of Veterinary Emergency and Critical Care; Steffen Professor of Veterinary Medicine, Department of Clinical Sciences, Section of Large Animal Medicine, Cornell University College of Veterinary Medicine, Ithaca, New York, USA

JEREMIAH EASLEY, DVM
Diplomate, American College of Veterinary Surgeons; ACVS Founding Fellow, Large Animal Minimally Invasive Surgery, Co-Director, Preclinical Surgical Research Laboratory, Assistant Professor, Department of Clinical Sciences, Translational Medicine Institute, Veterinary Teaching Hospital, Colorado State University, Fort Collins, Colorado, USA

DAVID E. FREEMAN, MVB, PhD
Diplomate, American College of Veterinary Surgeons; Appleton Endowed Professor, Equine Surgery, University of Florida, College of Veterinary Medicine, Large Animal Clinical Sciences, Gainesville, Florida, USA

DEREK C. KNOTTENBELT, BVM&S, DVM&S, MRCVS
Diplomate, European College of Equine Internal Medicine; Diplomate, American College of Veterinary Internal Medicine; Consultant in Equine Oncology, Equine Medical Solutions, Stirling, Scotland, United Kingdom

GUY D. LESTER, BVMS, PhD
Diplomate, American College of Veterinary Internal Medicine (Large Animal Internal Medicine); Department of Large Animal Clinical Sciences, College of Veterinary Medicine, University of Florida, Gainesville, Florida, USA

ROBERT J. MACKAY, BVSc (Dist), PhD
Diplomate, American College of Veterinary Internal Medicine; Professor, Department of Large Animal Clinical Sciences, University of Florida, Gainesville, Florida, USA

MARGO L. MACPHERSON, DVM, MS
Diplomate, American College of Theriogenologists; Reproduction, Department Large Animal Clinical Sciences, College of Veterinary Medicine, University of Florida, Gainesville, Florida, USA

DIANNE McFARLANE, DVM, PhD
Diplomate, American College of Veterinary Internal Medicine; Professor and Ricks Rapp Professor of Equine Research, Department of Physiological Sciences, Center for Veterinary Health Sciences, Oklahoma State University, Stillwater, Oklahoma, USA

MARK MEIJER, DVM
Dierenkiniek Zeddam, Zeddam, The Netherlands

LYNN PEZZANITE, DVM, MS
Diplomate, American College of Veterinary Surgeons; Preclinical Surgical Research Laboratory, Department of Clinical Sciences, Translational Medicine Institute, Veterinary Teaching Hospital, Colorado State University, Fort Collins, Colorado, USA

KIRSTIE PICKLES, BVMS, MSc, PhD, CertEM(IntMed), MRCVS
Diplomate, European College of Equine Internal Medicine; Consultant in Equine Medicine, Chine House Veterinary Hospital, Sileby, Leicestershire, United Kingdom

MALGORZATA A. POZOR, DVM, PhD
Diplomate, American College of Theriogenologists; Department of Large Animal Clinical Sciences, College of Veterinary Medicine, University of Florida, Gainesville, Florida, USA

JOY E. TOMLINSON, DVM
Diplomate, American College of Veterinary Internal Medicine; Research Associate, Baker Institute for Animal Health, Cornell University College of Veterinary Medicine, Ithaca, New York, USA

RAMIRO E. TORIBIO, DVM, MS, PhD
Diplomate, American College of Veterinary Internal Medicine; Professor of Equine Internal Medicine, Department of Veterinary Clinical Sciences, College of Veterinary Medicine, The Ohio State University, Columbus, Ohio, USA

GERLINDE R. VAN DE WALLE, DVM, PhD
Associate Professor, Baker Institute for Animal Health, Cornell University College of Veterinary Medicine, Ithaca, New York, USA

ANDREW W. VAN EPS, BVSc, PhD
Associate Professor, Department of Clinical Studies - New Bolton Center, School of Veterinary Medicine, University of Pennsylvania, Kennett Square, Pennsylvania, USA

Contents

This article discusses the main treatments for sarcoid and the specific difficulties of these. It explains to some extent why the frustrations of a condition for which there is no single treatment option have led to the burgeoning of an industry of irrational treatments. The factors that need to be considered before selecting an option for treatment are wider than is the case in most other disease entities as a result of the complexity of the condition, its variable phenotypes, and the individual perceptions and experiences of both veterinarians and owners.

 Video content accompanies this article at http://www.vetequine. theclinics.com.

Horses with trigeminal mediated headshaking (TMHS) have a decreased activation threshold of the trigeminal nerve and clinical signs are suspected to be a manifestation of trigeminal neuralgia. Electrical nerve stimulation (ENS) is used for management of neuralgia in humans and appears to work via gate control theory. Use of an equine specific percutaneous ENS program in over 130 TMHS horses has resulted in approximately 50% success return to previous work. Electroacupuncture may also be useful in the management TMHS. Optimization of ENS procedures for TMHS is likely to require a greater understanding of the etiopathogenesis of the aberrant neurophysiology.

Intravenous lidocaine is widely used to prevent or treat postoperative ileus in horses. Clinical studies that support this approach are flawed and contradicted by others. Also, physical obstruction could be more important in causing postoperative reflux than postoperative ileus in the horse. The antiinflammatory properties of lidocaine and the role of inflammation from intestinal handling in the genesis of postoperative reflux are questionable. Because of cost and questionable efficacy of lidocaine, a well-designed clinical trial is required to support its continued use. However, lidocaine could be given to provide or enhance analgesia in selected cases with postoperative colic.

Retained fetal membranes are the most common postpartum condition in mares. Although the incidence of retained fetal membranes is low, the consequences for the health of the mare can be severe (metritis, endotoxemia, laminitis, death). Oxytocin administration is often the first line of therapy for management of retained fetal membranes. Removal of fetal membranes using umbilical vessel infusion and manual membrane removal are effective tools for reducing risks associated with abnormally heavy membranes, retained membranes, or for mares that are geographically limited for veterinary care.

Cervical vertebral compressive myelopathy (CVCM) represents the most significant disease of the spinal cord in horses for which surgical treatment is described. Current surgical methods used include ventral interbody fusion with kerf cut cylinders and dorsal laminectomy. Polyaxial pedicle screw and rod constructs and ventral locking compression plating have been introduced in the treatment of equine CVCM and present promising alternative approaches to achieve ventral interbody fusion. Advancements in diagnostic imaging and endoscopy of the cervical vertebral canal may improve reliable preoperative identification of the exact locations of spinal cord compression in horses with CVCM to improve postoperative outcomes.

All gray horses inherited a single gene mutation, $STX17^G$, that alters melanocyte behavior to cause graying and propensities to develop vitiligo and melanoma. The coat color genes $ASIP^a$ and $MC1R^E$ add risk such that relative likelihood of melanoma based on pregraying coat color is black > bay > chestnut. Melanomas begin at about 4 years. Locoregional control of melanoma masses depends on surgical removal and/or intralesional chemotherapy (possibly with adjunctive hyperthermia or electroporation). Systemic treatment is not evidence based but immunomodulators (cimetidine, levamisole) and vaccines can be tried.

Despite there being only 2 common endocrine diseases in horses, pituitary pars intermedia dysfunction (PPID) and equine metabolic syndrome (EMS), diagnosis is still confusing. Failing to consider horse factors and treating based on laboratory results only have caused many animals to receive lifelong drug treatment unnecessarily. Increased plasma ACTH, baseline or TRH stimulated, supports a diagnosis of PPID; however, breed, age, thriftiness, illness, coat color, geography, diet, and season also affect ACTH concentration. Insulin dysregulation, the hallmark of EMS, can result from insulin resistance or excessive postprandial insulin release. Each requires a different diagnostic test to reach a diagnosis.

Exercise-induced pulmonary hemorrhage (EIPH) occurs commonly in horses undergoing strenuous exercise. Reported risk factors include racing in cold temperatures and wearing of bar shoes. In horses with documented moderate to severe EIPH, increasing the interval between races and adopting a negative race pace strategy may reduce the severity of EIPH in subsequent races. EIPH seems to have an impact on performance only when moderate to severe. This occurs in a small number of starters, approximately 6%. EIPH often is erratic in severity from race to race, although across a population it is weakly progressive over increasing race starts.

Theiler disease (serum hepatitis or idiopathic acute hepatic necrosis) has long been suspected to have a viral etiology. Four viruses have been described in association with hepatitis in horses. Further investigation suggests equine pegivirus and Theiler disease–associated virus (a second pegivirus) are neither hepatotropic nor pathogenic. Nonprimate hepacivirus (NPHV) causes subclinical disease in experimental models and has been associated with hepatitis in some clinical cases. Equine parvovirus-hepatitis (EqPV-H) experimentally causes subclinical-to-clinical liver disease and is found in the vast majority of Theiler disease cases. EqPV-H is likely of clinical significance, whereas the significance of NPHV is unknown.

Neonatal encephalopathy (NE) and neonatal maladjustment syndrome (NMS) are terms used for newborn foals that develop noninfectious neurologic signs in the immediate postpartum period. Cerebral ischemia, hypoxia, and inflammation leading to neuronal and glial dysfunction and excitotoxicity are considered key mechanisms behind NE/NMS. Attention has been placed on endocrine and paracrine factors that alter brain cell function. Abnormal steroid concentrations (progestogens, neurosteroids) have been measured in critically ill and NE foals. In addition to supportive treatment, antimicrobials should be considered. Controversies regarding the pathophysiology, diagnosis, and treatment of NE and NMS will remain until controlled mechanistic and therapeutic studies are conducted.

Laminitis is a consequence of primary disease processes elsewhere in the body. The key pathophysiologic events are insulin dysregulation in endocrinopathic laminitis, ischemia in supporting limb laminitis, and inflammation in sepsis-related laminitis. These apparently disparate mechanisms converge to cause lamellar attachment failure through epithelial cell adhesion loss and stretch, possibly mediated by common growth factor signaling pathways. Tissue damage through mechanical distraction, inflammation, pain, and a proliferative epithelial healing response are features of acute laminitis regardless of the cause. Preventive and treatment strategies based on knowledge of these unique and common mechanistic events are likely to improve clinical outcomes.

VETERINARY CLINICS OF NORTH AMERICA: EQUINE PRACTICE

RELATED SERIES

Veterinary Clinics of North America: Food Animal Practice

THE CLINICS ARE NOW AVAILABLE ONLINE!
Access your subscription at:
www.theclinics.com

VETERINARY CLINICS OF
NORTH AMERICA: EQUINE PRACTICE

Preface

And Now for Something Completely Different: Some Controversies in Equine Medicine, Surgery, and Reproduction

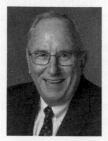

Robert J. MacKay, BVSc (Dist), PhD
Editor

It has been an honor and privilege to be able to recruit distinguished authors from among multiple disciplines to contribute to this issue and to superintend their manuscripts through to publication. The process has been an unusual challenge as this issue is not primarily a series of state-of-the-art reviews, as is the usual custom. Rather, with the help and advice of consulting editor, Tom Divers, I have for each article selected an element of a topic that is controversial, not universally agreed upon, or otherwise unclear. The purpose is to analyze the available evidence through the lens of each author's special expertise in order to provide some definition and clarity to the topic or at least explode a few myths. The first 6 articles are about effectiveness of certain treatments; the next one deals with diagnosis; then 2 articles make arguments as to the importance (or not) of the particular topic, and the final 2 articles explore controversial aspects of pathophysiology.

I hope some of the questions addressed in these articles will resonate with readers. Thumbnail questions are summarized here in the order they appear in the table of contents. Sarcoid is the most common cutaneous tumor of equids, but many treatments lack rationale or evidence of effectiveness. Have molecular and technical innovations led to progress in treatment? *Knottenbelt*. Head shakers are easy to diagnose but notoriously difficult to treat. Will some version of transcutaneous electrical nerve stimulation (TENS) provide a reliable and long-term solution? *Pickles.* Following small intestinal surgery, it is common practice to infuse lidocaine to prevent or treat ileus. Is postoperative ileus an important problem, and, if so, is lidocaine effective therapy? *Freeman.* Extraction of retained fetal membranes is not straightforward. Is there a

Vet Clin Equine 35 (2019) xi–xii
https://doi.org/10.1016/j.cveq.2019.05.001
0749-0739/19/© 2019 Published by Elsevier Inc.

simple and effective way to do it? *Burden, Meijer, Pozor, and Macpherson*. Interbody vertebral fusion is a well-established but lightly used treatment for wobblers that is performed now much as it was in the 1980s. Is there anything new on the horizon? *Pezzanite and Easley*. Grayness and melanomas of horses are genetically linked. Is there an effective way to manage these tumors? *MacKay*. Seasonally adjusted reference ranges, effects of stress and feeding on results, stimulations versus constitutive values: Can endocrine disorders be reliably diagnosed? *McFarlane*. There is now a wealth of epidemiologic analyses relating to exercise-induced pulmonary hemorrhage (EIPH). Are conclusions based on these data definitive, and is there consensus on the clinical consequences of EIPH? *Crispe*. News of scary-sounding hepatitis viruses has burst onto the scene, but are these viruses a serious threat? *Tomlinson, Van de Walle, Divers*. Theories as to the cause or causes of dummy foals seem to have dichotomized into perinatal deprivation versus endocrine immaturity. Can these both be right, and, if so, what is the relationship between the 2 theories? *Toribio*. Most readers have seen sophisticated diagrams showing networks of mediators and events underlying each of the laminitis types, namely, sepsis-associated, endocrinopathic, and (to a lesser extent) supporting limb. Do these networks overlap, and are there implications for prevention and treatment? *Van Eps and Burns*.

Finally, I would like to thank all the authors for their excellent contributions, and Tom Divers and the staff at Elsevier for their help in putting this issue together.

Robert J. MacKay, BVSc (Dist), PhD
Large Animal Clinical Sciences
University of Florida
PO Box 100136
Gainesville, FL 32610, USA

E-mail address:
mackayr@ufl.edu

The Equine Sarcoid
Why Are There so Many Treatment Options?

Derek C. Knottenbelt, BVM&S, DVM&S, MRCVS

KEYWORDS

- Sarcoid • Treatment • Chemotherapy • Surgery • Laser • Radiotherapy
- Immunotherapy

KEY POINTS

- The sarcoid continues to perplex and frustrate practicing veterinarians because there is no consistently effective treatment. This problem is complicated by the diversity of the phenotype of the lesions associated with it.
- Treatment considerations include the type of tumor present, its location, the extent and duration of the lesion, and that the condition is often belittled and subjected to ill-advised, often harmful treatment attempts.
- In addition, the logistics of treatment and the financial aspects of the treatment options challenge clinicians and widen the need for simple, basic, and effective treatments.
- All treatments have significant implications in some practical or financial aspects.

INTRODUCTION

The equine sarcoid is by far the commonest cutaneous neoplasm of horses, and the risk factors that predispose to its development in individuals have only partially been identified.[1] It affects horses of all ages, although most cases are first presented between 2 and 9 years of age. Sex seems to play no significant role, although there have been suggestions that geldings are overrepresented. Almost all breeds of horse, mule, donkey, and zebra are susceptible.

Historically the condition has been managed by individual veterinarians in ways that they find effective, or at least as effective as they are prepared to accept, which has led to many anecdotal reports and many short series of retrospective cases and to a wide variety of more or less effective treatment options. The problem is the absence of meaningful prospective double-blinded trials for many of the current treatments, and this has severely hampered the development of its treatment. It has also driven a whole industry of irrational and often dangerous interferences. A simple scan of

Disclosure: The author is Director of Equine Medical Solutions, a company providing advice and treatments for equine oncology patients.
Equine Medical Solutions Ltd, STEP Building, Kildean Business & Enterprise Hub, 146 Drip Road, Stirling, Scotland, FK8 1RW, UK
E-mail address: knotty@liverpool.ac.uk

Vet Clin Equine 35 (2019) 243–262
https://doi.org/10.1016/j.cveq.2019.03.006
0749-0739/19/© 2019 Elsevier Inc. All rights reserved.

vetequine.theclinics.com

the Internet reveals countless reports of the 100% successful treatment of this distressing and dangerous disease. These reports include the idiotic application of toothpaste or turmeric paste and turmeric in feed supplements, topical applications of salves, and sundry witchdoctor-type managements, all of which are based on the success of 1 or a few cases that seem to have resolved when subjected to a particular approach. Such reports often induce a hysterical response from owners with affected horses: anything that avoids veterinary consultation is viewed as worth trying. This approach probably accounts for a large number of different treatments used across the world.

It is a matter of considerable regret that the condition is generally viewed by owners as a virus infection rather than a neoplastic condition, and this has then fueled a desire to administer supposedly immune stimulating herbs and salts. This concept has to some extent been enhanced by the investigations into the etiopathogenesis of the disease. The relationship to the bovine papilloma virus (BPV) is still poorly understood, and the lack of any successful vaccination program for the BPV in the management or prevention of this disease has not led to a better understanding among horse owners that the sarcoid is a form of skin cancer. Most owners view the disease as a cosmetic nuisance and so many cases are presented in an advanced state having had multiple irrational interferences. If any of these interferences results in an apparently successful outcome, within hours the social media dissemination results in a dramatic bias toward that particular approach. Clinicians need to protect horses from this type of approach by ensuring that their understanding of the disease and their management of it are exemplary and take account of the neoplastic nature of the condition.

The easy answer to the question "Why are there so many treatments for the equine sarcoid?" is simply that there are no consistently reliable treatments for every type of sarcoid in every location in every horse and under all conditions (**Fig. 1**).

The choice of treatment or management is influenced by individual experience and several other factors (**Box 1**).

The Type of Sarcoid

The type of sarcoid involved and the specific pathologic characteristics and behavior of the individual sarcoid lesions in each horse need to be identified (see **Fig. 1**). Six different types of sarcoid have been identified, with some of these having subtypes that influence the treatment options available[2] (**Fig. 2**). It is important to point out that individual lesions of different sarcoid types often require very different treatments. In addition, there is often an inexplicable variation in response to individual treatments even when the lesions look ostensibly the same and are situated in broadly the same anatomic region. The same treatment can also bring different results when used by different veterinarians. What works for one may not work for another.

The Anatomic Location of the Sarcoid

Sarcoids in different locations seem to have different clinicopathologic characteristics (See **Fig. 1**). Sarcoids around the eye tend to be very invasive with penetration into the underlying diffuse musculature.[3] The upper eyelid is clearly more important than the lower eyelid in terms of the treatment options; damage to an upper eyelid can be critical and create severe functional compromise, whereas those on the lower eyelid tend to create little functional problem but have a significant cosmetic implication. Sarcoids overlying branches of the facial nerve or over joints are more challenging and the therapeutic options are correspondingly narrower and more problematic. Sarcoids occurring on the ear tend to remain firmly localized. Possibly the most dangerous of all sites

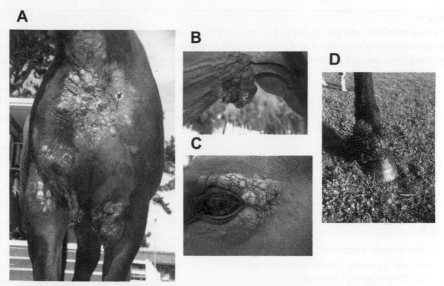

Fig. 1. The equine sarcoid is unique in respect of its causes and its epidemiology. It also occurs in 6 distinct forms and individual animals may have several or many lesions, which may be varied in appearance and location. Clinicians need to make sensible, practical, and defensible therapeutic decisions based on published evidence and experience. What works for one veterinarian does not always work for another. Not every treatment is available, practicable, or affordable in every clinical circumstance. This disease demands careful consideration because the wrong decision can result in a catastrophic outcome. Therapy has to be directed first at destroying the tumor in its entirety. The last cell is the most important one. The second objective is to preserve function. Cosmesis is an incidental aspect from a medical viewpoint but is often an overriding aspect for owners. (*A*) Multiple extensive verrucose sarcoids with a long history of continued progression and multiple ill-advised interventions. Any management here would have to be on a palliative basis. (*B*) This multifocal fibroblastic sarcoid in the midline anterior to the mammary region developed over a 12-month period from a single fly bite; this is a common owner-reported progression. Treatment of this lesion would require careful thought and the prognosis would usually be positive, if guarded, so long as the right clinical/therapeutic decisions were made on first presentation. (*C*) Eyelid sarcoids have particular therapeutic challenges and many of the conventional treatments are contraindicated because eyelid function damage can have serious outcomes. (*D*) A fibroblastic sarcoid on the pastern region that developed at the site of a small nonhealing wound.

for sarcoid development are the point of the elbow and the side of the face; for some reason there is a much greater tendency for local invasion and transformation to malignant sarcoid in these locations (**Fig. 3**). At these sites in particular, and perhaps to a lesser extent around the eye, sarcoid treatment is severely curtailed by the behavior of the tumor in particular sites. Where the sarcoid overlies bone, such as over the nasal or maxillary region, there are additional constraints and often major variations in treatment options. Combination therapies are often required.

Even where lesions look the same and are situated in broadly the same anatomic area there may be variations in the responses to individual treatments. The reasons for this are unknown but practitioners will recognize the pattern. The conclusion here is that the location is a fundamental factor to consider when making clinical therapeutic decisions. The wrong choice of the wrong treatment at the wrong time in the wrong place can have catastrophic outcomes. Treatments often need to be modified

Box 1
Factors that influence the choice of treatment of the equine sarcoid. Superimposed on this list is the overriding experience and facility available to individual veterinarians, who have varying facilities and experiences and what works for one may not work for another

1. Sarcoid type
2. Sarcoid location
3. Sarcoid extent
4. Sarcoid duration
5. Previous interference?
6. Prognosis
7. Logistics of treatment
8. Relative value of horse
9. Relative cost of treatment
10. Duration of treatment
    a. Management of treatment process
    b. Time to return to work
11. Animal compliance
12. Owner compliance

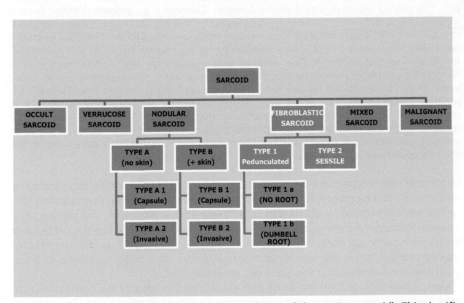

Fig. 2. A suggested classification of the common forms of the equine sarcoid). This classification matters because therapy for each type will necessarily be different. In addition, there are constraints in respect of treatment from location and extent. (*Adapted from* Knottenbelt DC. A suggested clinical classification for the equine sarcoid. Clin Tech Equine Pract 2006; 4, 278–95; with permission.)

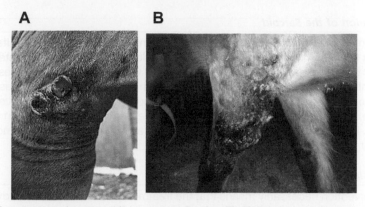

Fig. 3. The anatomic location of the sarcoid can be significant from both prognostic and therapeutic aspects. Sites such as the elbow (as shown here), the eyelid, and prefemoral flank fold have a high rate of invasion and a greater tendency to local malignancy. This relatively benign tumor (*A*) developed rapidly into a life-threatening invasive complex in the olecranon region. (*B*) Treatment will be highly problematic.

and combined therapies need to be chosen. What works on the flank is unlikely to be tolerated on the eyelid. Similarly, what works on an eyelid could be too weak for a lesion on the sheath or medial thigh.

The Extent and Number of Sarcoids

Small localized tumors are easier to treat and have a wider range of options (**Fig. 4**). Extensive tumors inevitably have limited options available, although, with patience and care, and sensible use of the available treatments, significant benefits can be achieved. Clearly this category of limitation is strongly related to the type of sarcoid and its anatomic location.

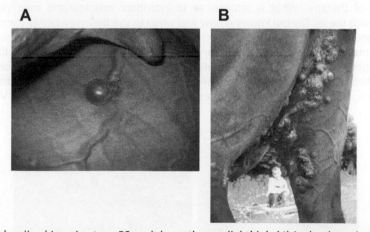

Fig. 4. A localized invasive type B2 nodule on the medial thigh (*A*) is clearly easier to treat than multiple extensive nodules, as shown on the right (*B*). Additional therapeutic complications are shown by these 2 cases. The lesion on the left involves a large blood vessel. Note that the proximal vein is much bigger than the vein approaching the lesion. The lesion is invasive and fast growing. It needs urgent treatment. Any topical application to the lesion on the right would "kiss" onto the other side and cause serious collateral damage and therapeutic dilution on the treated side, which alters the choice of treatments.

The Duration of the Sarcoid

The pathologic behavior of individual sarcoid lesions varies markedly from site to site and from horse to horse. Since the sarcoid is widely viewed as an incidental, trivial cosmetic nuisance, veterinarians are usually faced with more advanced cases, which clearly influences the choice of treatments and the consequent prognosis. The concept of early intervention needs to be better understood by owners and veterinarians alike. Early intervention and persistence is an essential philosophy when treating sarcoids. Less severe treatments are required for earlier, less advanced tumors (see **Figs. 3** and **4**).

Previous Interventions

Prior intervention necessarily means that the treatment choice, however ill-advised or relevant/appropriate, has failed (**Fig. 5**). Recurrence following any interference with sarcoid is recognized as a major cause of exacerbation. Owners (and regrettably some veterinarians) may have attempted irrational or partial treatment without appropriate planning. In addition, traumatic injury to sarcoid is also known to cause exacerbation and this inevitably makes the choice of treatment more problematic.[1] A standard principle of cancer therapy is that it is easier, and more effective, to treat small isolated early tumors. This concept regrettably is not widely understood by horse owners, who usually consult the Internet long before they consult a veterinarian. The vast array of irrational treatments used worldwide makes it hard to identify the genuinely successful ones. A few studies have identified methods that work for particular types and locations of tumor,[3,4] but there is an inherent unpredictability about the condition in general that reflects the wide variety of placative or panic treatment choices that are often applied.

The Facilities Available and the Expertise of the Attending Veterinarian

Facilities, treatment availability, and statutory regulation all combine to limit the choices of therapy. What is accessible to individual veterinarians may vary, and even having the facility but knowing how and when to use them is a highly variable factor to consider. For example, radiation is the gold standard for treatment of periocular sarcoid but this is not widely available. Within the category of radiotherapy there are several options again, including variation in the method of delivery (plesiotherapy, brachytherapy, and teletherapy) and the type of radiation (electrons, gamma radiation, or X-rays). Again, combinations of these can be used in particular cases. Very few

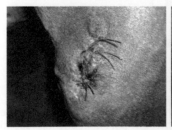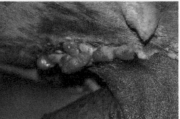

Fig. 5. Recurrence following a surgical treatment attempt (*left*) and a laser surgical excision (*right*). The recurrence following surgery is very rapid, whereas the recurrence following laser surgery is slower and is associated in this case with root recurrences. The choices for subsequent treatment become very narrow in this circumstance and combination treatment might have given a better result.

facilities exist for this treatment worldwide and so, although it is undoubtedly very effective in most cases (see **Fig. 2**), its overall value to clinicians is limited.

The most available method of treatment is surgery of one form or another. Again, within that choice there are multiple methods that can be used. Sharp surgery is the standard approach to sarcoid removal, but again the method can be limited in applicability by the type, location, duration, and extent of the sarcoid. A localized type A1 nodule is a good candidate for surgery on its own, but a severely invasive axillary sarcoid is probably not unless this can be combined with some adjunctive methods, including cryosurgery, chemotherapy, or even irradiation. Cryosurgery either on its own or with concurrent chemotherapy can be effective but, like all surgical methods, failure is common. Most publications relating to the surgical removal of sarcoid lesions give a prognostic figure of between 20% and 80% success; this in itself adds to the dilemma of whether to take a case to surgery or not. It is not possible to give an owner a true estimate of prognosis and most are not impressed by a realistic statement that recurrence can occur in between 80% and 20% of cases. Individual surgeons can improve their success rates by careful case selection.

Since seeding of the operative site with cells desquamated from the surface or roots of the tumor is an important cause of recurrence following surgery, efforts to reduce this are important. Laser, harmonic scalpel, or plasma knife technology help enormously, and again prognosis can be improved using these methods. Smart surgery is a method of minimal contamination surgery that is widely used in other species and can improve the rate of success of a surgical approach, particularly if combined with laser or harmonic scalpel instruments.[1]

Ligation of isolated lesions can be successful if the lesion is genuinely localized. Castration bands, elastic bands, and other ligatures have been used with variable success. Again, these ligation systems can be usefully combined with intralesional and topical chemotherapy. Systemic or topical chemotherapy demands special precautions and facilities.[5]

Owner and Horse Compliance

First, the horse must be able to tolerate the selected treatments. Some treatments are painful and others require general anesthesia, which may not be either wise or available. Repeated painful interventions may make the horse resistant to treatment. For example, treatment of an ear sarcoid with imiquimod results in severe pain and often major resentment so that the full course cannot be completed, and this in turn biases the treatment toward failure. Selection of a milder approach might simply mean failure from the outset. A further variable is the specific requirements and constraints placed by owners themselves. Financial aspects and logistic difficulties are often important factors that make the selection of treatment problematic. One owner might be more willing to accept an expensive treatment than another or may be willing to engage in a significant logistic process. Ultimately the owner has the final word after all the information has been provided; only then can an adequate informed decision be taken on what treatment to use.

The Relative Cost of the Treatment and the Patient

If the treatment costs more than the horse is worth, treatment choices may narrow; clearly this is variable. Emotional attachment to horses is common and so pure commercial value is then easily sidelined. Of course, owners want a cheap treatment but, in cancer medicine, a cheap treatment is not necessarily, or even usually, the best option. Cost should not be the primary concern unless particular circumstances exist for the owner. There is nothing more expensive than a cheap treatment that does not work, except of course an expensive treatment that does not work. Just because a treatment is cheaper it does not mean it is not good; indeed, there are plentiful treatments for sarcoids that are economical and effective. The most expensive treatment is probably irradiation (**Fig. 6**) but, because that is the gold standard for treatment of sarcoid, it could (if available) be justified on clinical grounds in most cases.

The ideal or best option treatment can be strongly influenced by several factors, and most of these are the same as the major considerations shown in **Box 1**. For example, radiation brachytherapy could be the best choice for a periocular diffuse invasive verrucose sarcoid but the facility may not be available or may cost too much for the owner and the horse may not travel well, so getting the horse to the facility may be a challenge. All of the factors shown in **Box 1** need to be considered in every case, and additionally there may be individual lesions on a horse that cannot tolerate the same treatment as might be effective or even ideal in another site. For example, a localized occult/mixed lesion on the medial thigh, as shown in **Fig. 3**, could justifiably be removed surgically, whereas a similar one situated over the parotid region origin of the facial nerve has very different demands.

It is important to realize that there are no boundaries in this decision process; clinicians need to be aware of all the factors that need to be considered and then try to match these with the available and affordable treatment options. Since there are plentiful therapy options, and even more combinations of treatment options, the choice is usually difficult. It is wise to consider carefully before embarking on a convenient option; it might not be the best (see **Fig. 5**). The individual factors are all interrelated to greater or lesser degree. No two cases, indeed probably no two lesions, are necessarily the same and clinical decision making needs to be subtle. If combinations of treatments are included in the available treatments for sarcoid, the number of options increases dramatically; as with many cancer conditions, combination therapy is commonly used (and should be) in the management of sarcoid. For example, following surgery, radiation, immunotherapy, intralesional and topical treatments are likely to improve the prognosis significantly.

The number of treatments used for sarcoid continues to climb, which suggests that clinicians are badly in need of a better overall treatment strategy and a greater understanding of the pathophysiology of the disease. As soon as therapeutic weakness is evident, the owner of a horse with sarcoid disease is drawn to the weird, the charlatanistic, the mysterious, and the homeopathic magic approach. Although this is irrational and incomprehensible to clinicians, it is a fact of life for veterinarians in practice.

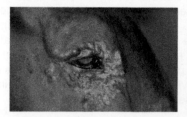 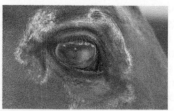

Fig. 6. This 14-year-old gelding was presented with extensive facial and periocular sarcoid of mixed type. It had received plentiful irrational therapy without success. Each attempt was accompanied by significant deterioration. Radiation brachytherapy resulted in a good outcome. Secondary effects including a focal cataract and corneal fibrosis were tolerated well and no recurrences were reported up to the euthanasia of the horse at 28 years of age for other reasons. The horse was lucky that the facilities existed and that the owner was prepared to cover the considerable expense. Both the horse and the owner were totally compliant and that made the process much simpler and more effective.

Ridiculous treatment options, including ligation with a tail hair, herbal feeds to boost immunity (whatever that means), the use of homeopathic diluted water, toothpaste, turmeric paste, tomatoes, and burnt toast are all used either prospectively before a veterinarian is consulted (usually as result of the ludicrous social media frenzy) or retrospectively when the veterinarian has failed to magically resolve the issue within a few days for no cost. Most of this irrationality is focused on the perception that a sarcoid is a wart and of trivial significance. The concept of cancer needs to be applied during all discussions with owners of affected horses. Frequent mention of the word cancer often brings owners to their senses, because that is what the disease is.

It is true to say that some irrational treatments do little harm, except that they delay the delivery of the appropriate treatment. However, most ill-advised interferences make the condition worse. Postinterference exacerbation is a well-recognized event in all cancer medicine and is particularly so for the equine sarcoid. Even biopsy can be a serious interference; a positive sarcoid diagnosis from a biopsy or partial excision should immediately trigger an effective treatment.

SO WHAT TREATMENT OPTIONS ARE THERE TO CHOOSE FROM?

Treatments for sarcoid can be broadly divided into categories of therapy and are shown in **Fig. 7**. Each of these categories have methods that have been assessed critically (usually retrospectively) but they also contain many other methods used and supported by individual veterinarians (and others) and anecdote. The common objective of all therapy is to remove every tumor cell and avoid seeding of the surgical site with cells that may survive and produce a new tumor. Failure to remove

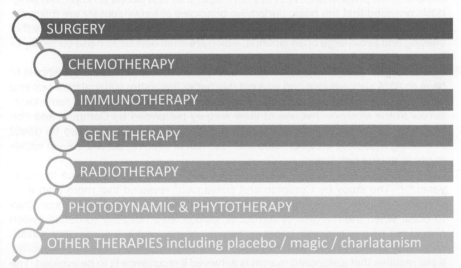

SURGERY

CHEMOTHERAPY

IMMUNOTHERAPY

GENE THERAPY

RADIOTHERAPY

PHOTODYNAMIC & PHYTOTHERAPY

OTHER THERAPIES including placebo / magic / charlatanism

Fig. 7. More than 40 different treatments and treatment combinations are described, but these can be broadly broken down into a smaller number of defined categories of treatment. Combinations and additional measures can also be used. For example, radiotherapy can be used after surgical tumor reduction and chemotherapy can be used to reduce the size of a tumor so that surgery becomes a feasible option. The large number of treatments available probably indicates that no single method is universally applicable to all sarcoid cases. In addition, there are severe constraints on what is useful or practicable in the clinical circumstances. Many treatments are limited in availability, so veterinarians need to make compromises.

every cell is usually a serious issue with sarcoid, no matter what treatment option is used, because of the characteristic invasive and diffuse margins. It is likely that the only totally effective way of removing every single cancer cell (in all neoplastic disease situations, not just sarcoid) is an induced immunologic response. Since this is the target of all oncological management in all species, it is unlikely that the equine sarcoid will be the first cancer to bring this outcome to a clinical conclusion. Extrapolation from other species is an inevitable part of the progress toward a cure.

Surgical Methods

1. Sharp surgical excision: all surgeons have their own records of success and/or failure with removal of sarcoids by surgical means. The basic concepts of surgical oncology are firstly to remove the tumor in its entirety and then avoid seeding into the operative site during the procedure. Of course, definition of a safe margin is tumor-type specific, with some tumors having clearly defined margins and others being much more invasive and harder to define. In sarcoid surgery the extent of the tumor is often impossible to define. Martens and colleagues[6] found that 33% of sarcoids excised with a margin of 1.6 cm had an unsafe margin (as shown by polymerase chain reaction detection of BPV). Closure and cosmesis are secondary but important concerns for an oncologic surgeon. In all cases the surgeon must try to achieve a safe margin and, if subsequent surgical pathology reveals an unsafe margin, concurrent measures, including wider excision, concurrent or adjunctive chemotherapy, or immunotherapy, must be instigated. The high rate of surgical failure in sarcoid surgery then promotes the use of diathermy or laser surgery but these are also problematic. They are not magic; they can deliver an improved prognosis provided that the basic underlying principles of tumor surgery are followed. Minimal contamination (smart) surgery can sometimes help to reduce the threat of seeding and avoid large open wounds, which are often difficult to close surgically or heal very slowly.[1]
2. Electrosurgical (diathermy) excision: in a recent study this approach was shown to have an 85% success rate and was notably better than other surgical methods and other chemotherapy approaches. The outcome of this study was remarkably similar to the study on the use of laser surgery performed by Compton and colleagues.[7] As an aside, harmonic scalpels and plasma knives can also be useful in creating bloodless surgical fields with less risk of seeding but are not yet widely in use in equine practice.
3. Laser excision: laser surgical removal of sarcoid lesions has been used for many years.[8–10] The study by Compton and colleagues[7] revealed that more than 80% of lesions resolved following laser surgical removal. Recurrence was more likely to occur when the margins of verrucose lesions were not easy to define, which should not be any surprise. Laser surgery is not magic; it is a surgically sophisticated way of ensuring a bloodless field with a very accurate excisional capability. It still requires that a standard margin is achieved if recurrence is to be avoided. The main advantage of laser surgery is the freedom from seeding of the operative site during the surgery and the ability to sterilize the wound bed after excision has been completed. An additional advantage is that the thermal injury extends the margin by a variable amount. CO_2 lasers leave less thermal injury than diode lasers so again there is a subtle difference in the surgical requirements for the two methods within this category. The disadvantages of laser surgery are the high rate of wound dehiscence if the wound site is closed primarily and the very slow healing process that is inherent in the method.

Laser surgery can be combined with various other treatments, including cryosurgery, local chemotherapy with slow release forms of carboplatin, cisplatin or 5-fluorouracil.

4. Ligation: ligation of the pedicle of pedunculated sarcoids or those sarcoids for which an artificial pedicle can be created by placement of an elasticated ligature around the tumor has been practiced for many years. The method works well provided that there is no extension of tumor below the ligature and can be combined with intralesional or topical chemotherapy. Obliteration of the blood supply to a tumor (however this is achieved) is a good if crude measure in oncology. Since this is an easy method to use, many owners do it themselves and they (and regrettably some veterinarians) can also apply idiotic ligation methods such as the use of tail hairs or suture material) around the neck of the lesion. As might be expected, these approaches are nonsensical and have a high rate of failure. Success is based more on luck than good judgment.

5. Cryosurgical ablation: cryosurgery causes necrosis of the tumor incorporated in the "ice ball." The method works reasonably well for superficial tumors but the ability of the horse to resist the cold is a major challenge. Restriction of blood flow during the procedure and the concurrent use of an intralesional or even topical chemotherapy agent such as 5-fluorouracil helps a great deal and, again, the restriction of blood flow during the procedure can give good results (**Fig. 8**). The procedure can be repeated until the site is tumor free and, because this is a nondemanding option, it is a valuable approach for practicing veterinarians. However, the margin is vital and typically the entire tumor must be necrotized along with a margin of safety. Since the method is nondiscriminatory and unpredictable, experience is valuable in the use of cryosurgical necrosis whether used with concurrent chemotherapy or not. The disadvantage is that there is no margin definition, and the success or failure is reflected in the presence or absence of recurrence. It is not always anatomically feasible or appropriate.

Chemotherapy

As might be expected with all cancer treatment, chemotherapy has to be a major consideration. Usually in the case of sarcoids, chemotherapy is applied either topically or intralesionally.

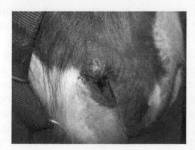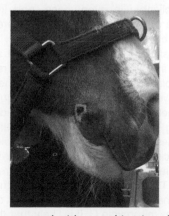

Fig. 8. This invasive type 2 fibroblastic sarcoid was treated with a combination of cryosurgery and local infiltration of 5-fluorouracil solution (50 mg/mL). Notice the extent of the secondary verrucose/occult changes around the lesion (*left*) and their complete disappearance once the sarcoid itself was treated (*right*).

1. Systemic chemotherapy: there are few reports of the use of systemic chemotherapy for sarcoid but it remains an attractive option for cases with very widespread sarcoid involvement. Only 1 study[5] has tested systemic chemotherapy against sarcoid disease and this showed that infusions of doxorubicin were an option that could be considered. It is likely that the constraints and restrictions of the use of doxorubicin in this report will restrict its use significantly. Nevertheless, it does hold promise for cases with very extensive tumors and specialist centers should be able to offer this as an option. Other combinations of more standard chemotherapy have not been tested but might also be applied in advanced cases.
2. Topical chemotherapy: a wide variety of topical treatments have been used. These range from antiviral agents such as acyclovir to antimitotic and cytotoxic or caustic applications.
   1. Acyclovir: a preliminary study by Stadler and colleagues[11] proposed treatment of small superficial sarcoid lesions with topical acyclovir. Publication of this study induced an almost hysterical demand for the method. Since acyclovir is widely used without prescription for herpes virus treatments in humans, lay owners opted for this treatment to avoid the need to consult veterinarians and a very high rate of failure and exacerbation resulted. Use of the material was irrational in many cases and a subsequent study revealed that it has little or no material benefit.[12] This is not surprising because the minor bystander effect on the suicide genes is extremely weak and would be unlikely to affect a robust mesenchymal tumor such as sarcoid.
   2. 5-Fluorouracil (5%) ointment: a commercially available ointment containing 5% 5-fluorouracil is widely used to treat superficial skin tumors in people. This material has also been shown to be an effective way of treating some superficial verrucose or occult sarcoid lesions. It can be used adjunctively with either cryosurgery or other surgical means and can have a good outcome.[3]
   3. AW5: this is a combination of fluorouracil, thiouracil, heavy metal salts, and steroid in a specially designed cream base that has been used by the author for more than 50 years with good effect. The material is restricted to veterinarians only. It is easy to apply but it is strictly controlled and treatment plans are devised specifically for individual tumors. Overall results depend on the type and extent of the sarcoids and the extent of previous treatment attempts, but nonrecurrence rates of around 74% are achievable.[1,13] It is not applicable in every case, and in particular is contraindicated around the eye or the side of the face where facial nerve or other critical damage can be caused.
3. Intralesional chemotherapy: several studies have been performed using intralesional injection of solutions or slow release emulsions or biodegradable implants of cisplatin. Intratumoral cisplatin chemotherapy was found to be a practical and effective treatment of sarcoid and squamous cell carcinoma/papilloma in horses.[14] Eighteen out of 19 horses with sarcoid lesions resolved. Biodegradable beads containing 1.6 mg of cisplatin (Matrix III, Wedgewood, Swedesboro, NJ) have also been tested in the treatment of sarcoids, usually as an adjunctive method to surgical excision.[15] In 11 out of 13 cases with sarcoid, animals were relapse free 2 years after treatment. Adverse effects were minimal and handling is relatively safe and easy. The use of slow release methods offers significant advantages compare with the use of aqueous solutions of chemotherapeutic drugs injected locally, such as mitomycin C. It is likely that the clearance of an aqueous solution is within minutes and this will limit the clinical benefit significantly unless blood flow can be restricted at least for a reasonable period.

4. Electrochemotherapy: several studies have identified that electrochemotherapy is a useful and effective way of treating sarcoid lesions of various types in various locations. The method is based on electrically induced increase in cell membrane permeability (electroporation) and the reported methods use either cisplatin or bleomycin. An in vitro study investigated the combined effects of electroporation and bleomycin, cisplatin, and carboplatin on an equine sarcoid cell line.[16] The use of electroporation increased the cytotoxic effects of bleomycin, cisplatin, and carboplatin on an equine sarcoid cell line in vitro by 5-fold, 4-fold, and 3-fold, respectively. These findings suggest that the in vivo effects of electroporation in sarcoid tumors can be useful in managing the disease. The method is versatile but does require repeated general anesthesia. Most cases respond after 4 to 6 treatments and some require up to 8.[17] Reported recurrence rates are low. Because any of several agents can be used, clinicians do have some choice in what is available. The author has used this with carboplatin and again good clinical resolution can be achieved with a simple process. Failures also occur, as might be expected.

5. Bleomycin: various attempts have been made to explore the efficacy of bleomycin in the treatment of sarcoid, including the use of electrochemotherapy and intralesional injection[16,18] with variable results. A recent pilot study by Knottenbelt and colleagues[19] identified that an ultradeformable liposomal preparation overcame at least some of the therapeutically inhibiting effects of endogenous bleomycin hydrolase enzymes; when used after pretreatment with either tazarotene or 5% 5-fluorouracil ointment the resolution rate was high (78%). The treatment was only used around the eye for defined verrucose or occult lesions but had singular advantages in being completely pain and inflammation free.

Immunotherapy

Since the discovery of the relationship between sarcoid tumors and BPVs[20] there have been determined attempts to identify immunologic methods of treatment. Clearly a therapeutic vaccination, or at least a preventive vaccination, would be the perfect solution. The problem is that it is a lot more complicated than this and vaccination for BPV does not prevent sarcoid development and neither do horses with sarcoid seroconvert to BPV. More sophisticated Immunologic methods are clearly required and much research is being dedicated to this objective, so far with little apparent positive practical and affordable benefit. Nevertheless, research continues and several reports of different immunologically based methods have been reported already. The search continues.

1. Spontaneous resolution. Throughout the history of sarcoid treatment, reports of spontaneous resolution have appeared. There is no doubt that a small proportion of sarcoids do resolve without treatment.[1,21,22] This resolution is a remarkable event involving the spontaneous and usually rapid self-cure of all sarcoids on a horse. There are also some cases in which an individual lesion seems to resolve spontaneously but others on the same horse do not. In the author's experience, horses that fully and rapidly self-resolve seem also to be solidly immune to the disease thereafter. Spontaneous resolution is seemingly less common in donkeys.

2. Immunomodulation using bacillus Calmette-Guérin (BCG) and other protein materials. Klein and colleagues[23] performed a randomized study comparing cryosurgery with the use of a lyophilized BCG and a purified protein derivative from BCG. This study showed an impressive 100% success with cryosurgery but 60% success in the live BCG bacillus group and 70% with the purified cell wall extract group.

Similar results had been reported previously.[3,24,25] Knottenbelt and Kelly[3] also showed that the freeze-dried BCG was effective around the eyelid region in more than 75% of cases. An earlier study by Klein[26] found that the sarcoids on the distal limb were less responsive; in the investigator's experience BCG treatment on the distal limb seems to result in significant exacerbation. Most of the studies involving the use of BCG have not fully classified the type of sarcoid being treated and variation in response might reflect variation in the type, extent/size, location, and duration of the tumor. Several other immunomodulating protein materials have also been used with variable success. Attempts to administer these materials to induce generalized systemic immune responses have also been made but seem to carry very low success rates.

3. Vaccines. Kinnunen and colleagues[27] treated 21 horses with sarcoid tumors by bioimmunotherapy using autogenous vaccines made from extirpated tumor tissue by polymerization. Four out of 12 horses showed recurrence but the rest are reported to have resolved permanently. The pathophysiology of this is unknown but mitochondrial events are possibly involved. Hainisch and colleagues[28] also studied the potential preventive and therapeutic effects of BPV-1 L1 virus-like particles in a dose-escalation vaccination trial but no further studies have been reported as yet.

4. Autoinoculation/autografting. Espy[29] described the use of autologous grafts of tumor tissue subjected to liquid nitrogen freezing. Caitlin and colleagues[30] performed this same procedure in 18 cases and reported a high level of improvement and client satisfaction. In addition, Rothacker and colleagues[31] reported the use of the autograft method with a 68% regression of tumor size and a 46% complication rate; it is hard to understand why this approach has not become the gold standard if it works so well. It is also hard to understand what the rationale or the mechanism for this might be and few other reports have been made on the value of the method. However, complications are reported. Considerable risks occur and this kind of approach is not often described for the treatment of any cancerous condition in any other species.

5. Hemotherapy. Brandt and colleagues[32] identified BPV DNA sequences in peripheral blood of sarcoid-affected horses and donkeys. This finding suggests that, similarly to the bovine situation, the peripheral blood could possibly act as a vehicle of viral dissemination. This possibility is suggested as the rationale behind the use of hemotherapy. The practice is used widely in Central America and involves the withdrawal of venous blood and its immediate intramuscular injection. There is no published study relating to this but anecdotal reports of high success rates are encountered.

Gene Therapy

1. Mediator-governed therapy: several different cell-mediator mechanisms have been proposed, including the use of interleukins and plasmid-based therapy options.[33] No clinical trials are reported as yet but because genetic bases are largely responsible for susceptibility to the disease and because spontaneous resolutions do occur without any obvious seroconversion, it seems likely that some mediators are possibly responsible for both failure to resolve and successful resolution.

2. Genetic manipulation therapy: there are a few research studies that have used aspects of genetic manipulation but so far none has resulted in a practical therapeutic option.[34,35]

Radiotherapy

1. Teletherapy: few reports of the value of teletherapy exist in horses but it is expected to be highly effective.[1,36]
2. Brachytherapy: brachytherapy using various radioactive isotopes, including radon, iridium[192], and gold[198], has become the gold standard treatment of sarcoid.[37] The first reports of its use were made in 1979[38] and subsequent studies using low-dose or high-dose brachytherapy have been uniformly impressive[3,36,39,40] (see **Fig. 6**).
3. Plesiotherapy: direct application of a radioactive wand/stick delivering electrons (beta radiation) derived from decaying strontium[90] is a possible treatment of very superficial sarcoid lesions of very limited size.[1] There are no reports of extensive studies on this; it is probably impractical in most circumstances.

Photodynamic Therapy

Although photodynamic therapy is described as a treatment of equine sarcoid, there are no reports of extensive studies relating to its use. Several articles have been published describing its use in individual or several cases in which significant benefits were reported.[41] The theoretic advantages of its use are in its focal nature and its precision.[1] The disadvantages include the need for specialist equipment and experience. Several photodynamic agents can be used, including variants of aminolevulinic acid and hyperacin.[42]

Adjunctive Therapy

1. Tazarotene: this is a retinoid gel (0.1%) that is used widely to treat human disorders of keratinization, including Darrier disease and psoriasis. It can be used to remove the secondary epidermal changes that often accompany sarcoid tumors.[1,3]

Phytotherapy

1. A double-blinded trial testing the use of an extract of the white mistletoe plant (*Viscum album australicus*) (IscadorP, Iscadore Ag, Germany) performed by Christen-Clottu and colleagues[43] showed that repeated local injection of this extract had a significant beneficial effect on a range of sarcoid lesions. The procedure was painful and slow but the benefits were clearly positive. Chernyshov and colleagues[44] showed that the extract had a significant immunomodulating effect in humans. No further studies of this material have been performed in horses.
2. Blood root/zinc chloride mixtures: various forms of this mixture are marketed commercially, with manufacturers claiming high nonrecurrence rates. The respective roles in the treatment of sarcoid played by the bloodroot (*Sanguinaria canadensis*) and the 15% to 30% zinc chloride are not defined. The immunomodulating effects of sanguinarine have been explored in depth but little is known about their antitumor effects in fibroblastic tumor types. Black salve is a topical escharotic compound containing the active component sanguinarine derived usually from *S canadensis*. It has been advertised as a natural treatment of human skin cancer and is currently used widely by horse owners wishing to avoid veterinary consultation for treatment of sarcoids; Internet reports of more than 100% success are common. A theoretic risk exists of black salve inducing epidemic life-threatening dropsy in people[45] but there are no reports of generalized side effects in horses. The irrational use of this material without veterinary consultation carries risks, and most of the growth in its use is caused by its ease of accessibility from online vendors, invariably marketed with claims that are not scientifically tested and more usually completely irrational. Clinical trials in this area are lacking, with most clinical data in the form of case reports

showing suboptimal therapeutic and cosmetic outcomes associated with its use. However, in vitro studies of sanguinarine suggest it causes indiscriminate destruction of healthy and cancerous tissue at doses higher than 5 μg, limiting its practical value in any species. It is vital that members of the public are aware of the potential effects and toxicity of commercial salve products. Veterinary prescription should be obligatory.

Other Methods

1. Hyperthermia: this has been used effectively to treat superficial and deep tumors in human oncology but there are no significant reports of its use in equine sarcoid treatment. One report exists that mentions the technique.[9] The author has used it in 3 cases without long-term benefit.
2. Herbal diets: these are widely publicized in advertising and social media forums where anecdotal reports of amazing results are frequently made. The rationality of these materials is highly questionable and, if they worked so well, why are they not subjected to appropriate scientific scrutiny? They rely on jargon and baffling scientific "logic" to give them credibility. In truth, they would probably seldom do any harm apart from delaying appropriate therapy.
3. Fluoride toothpaste/mouthwash: again, the anecdotal reports of high efficacy in very advanced cases are plentiful on social media. The high concentrations of fluorine are suggested as being antisarcoid. If only cancer medicine was as simple as this!
4. Turmeric paste or dietary turmeric: the basis for the use of topical and dietary turmeric is the anticancer effects of cumin, its active ingredient. This material is claimed to have incredible powers of healing with efficacy against a very wide range of human and veterinary disease. Its alleged superpower should, of course, be subjected to appropriate scientific scrutiny but there are plentiful articles published on its value in human cancer treatment. Nevertheless, it is not a method that can be recommended unless and until it is properly tested. Again, it probably does little harm apart from creating delays in delivery of proper treatment.
5. Homeopathic remedies are, unfortunately, often used to treat sarcoids but, because they do nothing apart from cost the owner significant amounts of money, the results remain disappointing. The biggest problem again is the delay that the approaches bring to the case. Because those who peddle these materials have a positive explanation for improvement, static states, or deterioration, delays are common following these approaches. Charlatanism should be deterred, not encouraged; cancer treatment requires sensible, evidence-based approaches. It is not magic and it never will be.

It is unwise to conclude that plant-based treatments of cancer and sarcoid in particular will never treat cases of sarcoid because certain natural medicines, including aloe vera, rosemary oil, and tea tree oil, have, anecdotally, been found to help a few cases. However, any material that treats almost any disease in almost any species must be viewed with a degree of skepticism: if only it were that simple! It is also important to know that, in some cases, application of remedies of various natural and homeopathic types have resulted in considerable exacerbation of the tumors. This exacerbation is probably more a property of the tumors being interfered with than any directly harmful effect of the remedy.

Benign Neglect

The last of the vast array of treatments and combinations of treatments used in the management of sarcoid is the benign neglect approach. Benign neglect does not

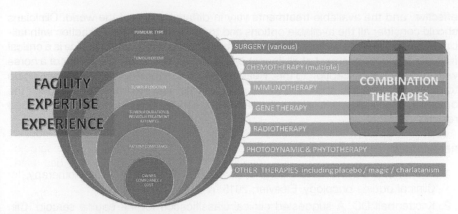

Fig. 9. Factors that influence the selection of treatment of equine sarcoid tumors. These factors are closely interrelated but form a basis for decision-making processes. Combination therapies are often used in oncological practice and this also applies to sarcoid, which explains at least partially why there are so many different variations and specific and nonspecific treatment options. Veterinary/surgical facilities and availability of specific methods add to the complexity of the decision. The relative size of the circle gives the relative importance of the feature. Superimposed over the decision-making process is the overriding concern that no harm should be done either by commission or by neglecting the disease.

mean neglect. In this case a clinical decision is made to leave the condition alone and to monitor it carefully. This approach is usually (but not always) made when the tumor is too far advanced for any practical treatment option, or when the tumor is very small and insignificant, or when the practicality/feasibility of other options is unacceptable. Palliative care of severe cases is sometimes unavoidable, although the patient welfare aspects of advanced disease need to be considered as the absolute priority. Some sarcoids remain static and clinically insignificant for years or even the whole life of the horse, but, again, it is important that the condition is monitored because the balance of probability is that the condition will develop in due course. In a few remarkable cases spontaneous remission occurs.[1,21,46] However, it is probably unwise to delay treatment on the off chance that the condition will undergo spontaneous remission.

SUMMARY

Almost countless treatments and combinations of treatments are used worldwide to treat this distressing and complex disorder (**Fig. 9**). Combinations of treatments add complexity to the process but, in so doing, the prognosis can also be significantly improved. Common sense and professionalism can be used to make clinical decisions that are relevant to the circumstance and provide the best available, convenient, and affordable treatment of a particular patient. Much of the treatment is irrational and, potentially at least, dangerous. It is far better in all probability to do nothing rather than to do harm by using irrational methods.

NOTHING is better than [just] SOMETHING especially if the SOMETHING is in fact not NOTHING

Possibly the major concern that clinicians have when faced with a case of sarcoid concerns what happens if the treatment fails. Will it get worse and will the clinician be blamed for that? The reality is that no treatment option is universally or totally effective, and the available treatments vary in different parts of the world. Clinicians should consider all the available options and try to establish a plan of action with fallback positions in the event of failure or incomplete responses. Client advice is a critical feature of the management of all cancer cases in all species, and the owner of a horse with sarcoid is no exception to this. Realism, pragmatism, understanding, keeping up to date, and a holistic approach to the case and not just the condition influence the outcome. From the wide array of treatments, sensible decisions can bring good results.

REFERENCES

1. Knottenbelt DC, Patterson Kane J, Snalune K. Principles of chemotherapy. In: Clinical equine oncology. Elsevier; 2015. p. 119–202.
2. Knottenbelt DC. A suggested clinical classification for the equine sarcoid. Clin Tech Equine Pract 2006;4:278–95.
3. Knottenbelt DC, Kelly DF. The diagnosis and treatment of periorbital sarcoid in the horse: 445 cases from 1974 - 1999. Vet Ophthalmol 2000;3:73–82.
4. Klein WR. Equine sarcoid immunotherapy. Practische Tierarzt 1988;69:17–8.
5. Théon AP, Pusterla N, Magdesian KG, et al. A pilot phase II study of the efficacy and biosafety of doxorubicin chemotherapy in tumor-bearing equidae. J Vet Intern Med 2013;27(6):1581–8.
6. Martens A, De Moor A, Demeulemeester J, et al. Polymerase chain reaction analysis of the surgical margins of equine sarcoids for bovine papilloma virus DNA. Vet Surg 2001;30(5):460–7.
7. Compston PC, Turner T, Wylie CE, Payne RJ. Laser surgery as a treatment for histologically confirmed sarcoids in the horse. Equine Vet J 2016;48(4):451–6.
8. Palmer SE. Carbon dioxide laser removal of a verrucous sarcoid from the ear of a horse. J Am Vet Med Assoc 1989;195(8):1125–7.
9. Marti E, Lazary S, Antczak DF, et al. Report of the first international workshop on equine sarcoid. Equine Vet J 1993;25(5):397–407.
10. Carstanjen B, Jordan P, Lepage OM. Carbon dioxide laser as a surgical instrument for sarcoid therapy–a retrospective study on 60 cases. Can Vet J 1997; 38(12):773–6.
11. Stadler S, Kainzbauer C, Haralambus R, et al. Successful treatment of equine sarcoids by topical aciclovir application. Vet Rec 2011;168(7):187.
12. Haspeslagh M, Jordana Garcia M, Vlaminck LEM, et al. Topical use of 5% acyclovir cream for the treatment of occult and verrucous equine sarcoids: a double-blinded placebo-controlled study. BMC Vet Res 2017;13(1):296.
13. Knottenbelt DC, Edwards SER, Daniel EA. The diagnosis and treatment of the equine sarcoid in Practice (supplement to Veterinary Record), vol. 17, 1995. p. 123–9.
14. Théon AP, Pascoe JR, Carlson GP, et al. Intratumoral chemotherapy with cisplatin in oily emulsion in horses. J Am Vet Med Assoc 1993;202(2):261–7.
15. Hewes CA, Sullins KE. Use of cisplatin-containing biodegradable beads for treatment of cutaneous neoplasia in equidae: 59 cases (2000-2004). J Am Vet Med Assoc 2006;229(10):1617–22.
16. Souza C, Villarino NF, Farnsworth K, et al. Enhanced cytotoxicity of bleomycin, cisplatin, and carboplatin on equine sarcoid cells following electroporation-mediated delivery in vitro. J Vet Pharmacol Ther 2017;40(1):97–100.

17. Tozon N, Kramaric P, Kos Kadunc V, et al. Electrochemotherapy as a single or adjuvant treatment to surgery of cutaneous sarcoid tumours in horses: a 31-case retrospective study. Vet Rec 2016;179(24):627.

18. Fürst, M. Klinische Studie über den Einsatz von Bleomycin bei der Behandlung von Equines Sarkoiden [Clinical evaluation of bleomycin for the treatment of equine sarcoid]. Inaugural-Dissertation zur Erlangung der Doktorwürde der Vet-suisse-Fakultät Universität Zürich Zurück zum Suchergebnis. 2006.

19. Knottenbelt DC, Watson AH, Hotchkiss JW, et al. A pilot study on the use of ultra-deformable liposomes containing bleomycin in the treatment of equine sarcoid. Equine Vet Educ 2018. https://doi.org/10.1111/eve.12950.

20. Reid SWJ, Reid KT. (1992) The equine sarcoid: Detection of papillomaviral DNA in sarcoid tumours by use of consensus primers and the polymerase chain reaction. Proceedings of the Sixth International Conference on Equine Infectious Disease, Cambridge, UK, 7–11 July 1991. p. 297-300.

21. Brostrom H. Equine sarcoids: a clinical, epidemiological and immunological study. Uppsala, Sweden: Swedish University of Agricultural Sciences; 1995. p. 33–9.

22. Goodrich L, Gerber H, Marti E. Equine Sarcoids. Veterinary Clinics of North America (Equine Practice) 1998;14:607–23.

23. Klein WR, Bras GE, Misdorp W, et al. Equine sarcoid: BCG immunotherapy compared to cryosurgery in a prospective randomised clinical trial. Cancer Immunol Immunother 1986;21(2):133–40.

24. Lavach JD, Sullins KE, Roberts SM, et al. BCG treatment of periocular sarcoid. Equine Vet J 1985;17(6):445–8.

25. Vanselow BA, Abetz I, Jackson AR. BCG emulsion immunotherapy of equine sarcoid. Equine Vet J 1988;20(6):444–7.

26. Klein WR. Immunotherapy of squamous cell carcinoma of the bovine eye and of equine sarcoid. Tijdschr Diergeneeskd 1990;115(24):1149–55.

27. Kinnunen RE, Tallberg T, Stenbäck H, et al. Equine sarcoid tumour treated by autogenous tumour vaccine. Anticancer Res 1999;19(4C):3367–74.

28. Hainisch EK, Brandt S, Shafti-Keramat S, et al. Safety and immunogenicity of BPV-1 L1 virus-like particles in a dose-escalation vaccination trial in horses. Equine Vet J 2012;44(1):107–11.

29. Espy BMK How to treat Equine sarcoids by autologous implants. Autologous grafting treatment for equine sarcoid. Proceedings of the American Association of Equine Practitioners AAEP 2008, 26–29 November 2000, San Antonio. 68-73.

30. Rothacker CC, Boyle AG, David G. Levine Autologous vaccination for the treatment of equine sarcoids: 18 cases (2009–2014). Can Vet J 2015;56(7):709–14.

31. Rothacker CC, Boyle AG, Levine DG. Autologous vaccination for the treatment of equine sarcoids: 18 cases (2009-2014). Can Vet J 2015;56(7):709–14.

32. Brandt S, Haralambus R, Schoster A, et al. Peripheral blood mononuclear cells represent a reservoir of bovine papillomavirus DNA in sarcoid-affected equines. J Gen Virol 2008;89:1390–5.

33. Mählmann K, Hamza E, Marti E, et al. Increased FOXP3 expression in tumour-associated tissues of horses affected with equine sarcoid disease. Vet J 2014; 202(3):516–21.

34. Gobeil PA, Yuan Z, Gault EA, et al. Small interfering RNA targeting bovine papillomavirus type 1 E2 induces apoptosis in equine sarcoid transformed fibroblasts. Virus Res 2009;145(1):162–5.

35. Yuan Z, Gault EA, Campo MS, et al. p38 mitogen-activated protein kinase is crucial for bovine papillomavirus type-1 transformation of equine fibroblasts. J Gen Virol 2011;92(Pt 8):1778–86.
36. Théon AP. Radiation therapy in the horse. Vet Clin North Am Equine Pract 1998; 14(3):673–88.
37. Théon AP, Pascoe JR. Iridium-192 interstitial brachytherapy for equine periocular tumours: treatment results and prognostic factors in 115 horses. Equine Vet J 1995;27(2):117–21.
38. Wynn-Jones G. Treatment of periocular tumours in horses using radioactive gold[198] grains. Equine Vet J 1979;11:3–5.
39. Byam-Cook KL, Henson FM, Slater JD. Treatment of periocular and non-ocular sarcoids in 18 horses by interstitial brachytherapy with iridium-192. Vet Rec 2006;159(11):337–41.
40. Hollis AR, Berlato D. Initial experience with high dose rate brachytherapy of peri-orbital sarcoids in the horse. Equine Vet Educ 2018;30:444–9.
41. Martens A, de Moor A, Waelkens E, et al. *In vitro* and *in vivo* evaluation of hyper-icin for photodynamic therapy of equine sarcoids the veterinary. Journal 2000; 159:77–84.
42. Buchholz J, Walt H. Veterinary photodynamic therapy: a review. Photodiagnosis Photodyn Ther 2013;10:342–7.
43. Christen-Clottu O, Klocke P, Burger D, et al. Treatment of clinically diagnosed equine sarcoid with a mistletoe extract (Viscum album austriacus). J Vet Intern Med 2010;24(6):1483–9.
44. Chernyshov VP, Heusser P, Omelchenko LI, et al. Immunomodulatory and clinical effects of Viscum album (Iscador M and Iscador P) in children with recurrent res-piratory infections as a result of the Chernobyl nuclear accident. Am J Ther 2000; 7(3):195–203.
45. Croaker A, King GJ, Pyne JH, et al. Assessing the risk of epidemic dropsy from black salve use. J Appl Toxicol 2018. https://doi.org/10.1002/jat.3619.
46. Berruex F, Gerber V, Wohlfender FD, et al. Clinical course of sarcoids in 61 Franches-Montagnes horses over a 5-7-year period. Vet Q 2016;36(4):189–96.

Is Electrical Nerve Stimulation the Answer for Management of Equine Headshaking?

Kirstie Pickles, BVMS, MSc, PhD, CertEM(IntMed), MRCVS

KEYWORDS

• Headshaking • Trigeminal • Neuromodulation • PENS • Electroacupuncture

KEY POINTS

• Trigeminal mediated headshaking is caused by a decreased threshold for activation of the trigeminal nerve in susceptible horses. Seasonal and spontaneous remission of headshaking suggests that this altered activation threshold may be reversible.

• Electrical nerve stimulation is useful for management of intractable pain syndromes and seems to work via gate control theory, whereby nociceptive information from small diameter afferents is overridden by the stimulation of large diameter fibers and activation of the descending inhibitory pathway.

• Use of an equine-specific percutaneous electrical nerve stimulation program in more than 130 horses has resulted in approximately 50% success in return to previous level of work for variable periods of time. A limited, small scale study has shown that electroacupuncture may also be useful in the management of headshaking.

• Other forms of electrical nerve stimulation such as implants are useful for long-term control of neuropathic pain in humans and warrant investigation in horses that respond to intermittent peripheral nerve stimulation.

• Optimization of electrical nerve stimulation procedures for the treatment of headshaking is likely to require a greater understanding of the pathophysiology of the aberrant trigeminal nerve function.

Video content accompanies this article at http://www.vetequine.theclinics. com.

INTRODUCTION

Trigeminal mediated headshaking (TMHS) is a spontaneously occurring disorder of mature horses characterized by violent, usually vertical, shakes, flicks, or jerks of the head, in the absence of any apparent physical stimulus.[1–3] Other clinical signs

Conflict of Interest Statement: The author has no commercial or financial conflicts of interest.
Chine House Veterinary Hospital, 12 Cossington Road, Sileby, Leicestershire LE12 7RS, UK
E-mail address: kpickles@chinehousevets.co.uk

Vet Clin Equine 35 (2019) 263–274
https://doi.org/10.1016/j.cveq.2019.03.002
0749-0739/19/© 2019 Elsevier Inc. All rights reserved.

include snorting, an "anxious" facial expression and muzzle rubbing, which can be so intense that horses strike at their nose with their thoracic limbs or inflict considerable self-trauma. Severely affected horses seem to have compromised welfare and can be dangerous to handle and ride due to their unpredictable behavior. TMHS seems to have a worldwide distribution and a prevalence of 4.6% has been reported in the United Kingdom[4]; therefore a significant number of horses are likely to be affected.

Despite the trigeminal nerve having long been implicated in the pathophysiology of TMHS due to the presenting clinical signs,[5] definitive involvement has only recently been confirmed. Detailed nerve conduction studies of control and headshaking horses have identified a reduced activation threshold of the trigeminal nerve in headshaking horses.[6] Intriguingly, approximately 60% of headshaking horses are seasonally affected with clinical disease present only in the spring, summer, and sometimes autumn months,[2,7] suggesting reversibility of any altered neurophysiology. The clinical signs of TMHS are suspected to be a manifestation of trigeminal neuropathic pain and the disease seems to share some clinical similarities with human trigeminal neuralgia (HTN). Sufferers of HTN report intermittent or continuous burning, itching, tingling, tickling, or electric shock–like pain originating in the areas innervated by the trigeminal nerve,[8] which seem to equate well to the observed signs displayed by horses with TMHS.

Current therapeutic options are limited by our incomplete understanding of this trigeminal nerve sensitization and its role in the etiopathogenesis of TMHS. It is also possible that there is more than one cause with the same clinical manifestation, leading to different response rates to treatment. However, newer therapies such as electrical nerve stimulation seem to offer a more rational approach to management of the disease. This paper reviews trigeminal nerve anatomy, the current knowledge of the etiopathogenesis of TMHS, and the evidence for use of electrical nerve stimulation in its management.

ANATOMY OF THE TRIGEMINAL COMPLEX

The trigeminal complex is formed of peripheral and central components. Peripheral components consist of the trigeminal nerve (V cranial nerve), trigeminal ganglion, the 3 main branches (ophthalmic, maxillary, mandibular [**Fig. 1**]), and subsequent branches. The central components comprise the spinal tract, which might extend

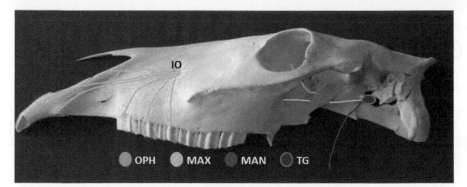

Fig. 1. Peripheral components of the trigeminal complex. Ophthalmic nerve (OPH in *green*), maxillary nerve (MAX and its branch infraorbital nerve [IO], in *yellow*), mandibular nerve (MAN in *red*), and trigeminal ganglion (oval brown structure). Not all branches from each nerve are shown. Figure not drawn to scale. (*From* Pickles K, Madigan J, Aleman M. Idiopathic headshaking: is it still idiopathic? Vet J. 2014 Jul;201(1):21–30; with permission.)

up to the second cervical spinal cord segment, and nuclei of the trigeminal complex within the brainstem.

The trigeminal nerve is the largest sensory cranial nerve and carries information relating to light touch, temperature, pain, and proprioception from the face and head to the brain. The sensory components include the ophthalmic, maxillary, and mandibular nerves.[9] The mandibular nerve also has motor function. The trigeminal ganglion contains sensory cell bodies for pain and temperature modalities of all 3 sensory nerves of the trigeminal nerve.[9]

The cell bodies of neurons of proprioceptive modalities are not located in the trigeminal ganglion but in nuclei within the brainstem.[9] The motor part of the mandibular nerve is ventral to the trigeminal ganglion. The ophthalmic nerve is the smallest of the 3 sensory nerves and runs lateral to the cavernous sinus. The ophthalmic nerve enters the orbital fissure along with the oculomotor, trochlear, abducens, and sympathetic nerves to the eye. The ophthalmic nerve gives rise to the lacrimal, frontal, nasociliary, and ethmoidal nerves.[10]

The maxillary nerve emerges from the round foramen and continues into the maxillary foramen and infraorbital canal as the infraorbital nerve. The maxillary nerve has several branches including the zygomaticofacial, pterygopalatine, major palatine, minor palatine, caudal nasal, and infraorbital nerves.[10] The caudal nasal nerve has been commonly referred to as the posterior ethmoidal nerve; however, these nerves are distinct structures arising from different branches of the trigeminal nerve. The mandibular nerve gives rise to (among others) the masseteric, temporal, pterygoid, tensor tympani, tensor veli palatini, mylohyoid, auriculotemporal, buccal, lingual, and mental nerves.[10] The signs of apparent facial discomfort displayed by affected horses seem to be mainly localized to the muzzle/nose area. The maxillary nerve is sensory to the lower eyelid, maxillary teeth, upper lip, maxillary sinus, and nose.

ETIOPATHOGENESIS OF TRIGEMINAL MEDIATED HEADSHAKING
Altered Trigeminal Neurophysiology

Recent neurophysiology studies[6,11] have demonstrated a significant difference in the threshold for activation of the infraorbital nerve, a branch of the maxillary division of the trigeminal nerve, between control and TMHS horses (**Fig. 2**). Affected horses have a significantly lower stimulus threshold ($\leq$5 mA) than control horses ($\geq$10 mA). Once a sensory action potential was triggered, there were no differences in any neurophysiologic parameters measured, including conduction velocity. In addition, there were no differences between left and right sides demonstrating bilateral involvement of the trigeminal nerve in affected horses and validating the bilateral clinical manifestations of the syndrome.

Interestingly, a horse with seasonal TMHS tested (only) during a time of remission showed a threshold for activation similar to control horses. This, and the seasonal nature of TMHS in more than half of affected horses, suggests that the threshold of the nerve is malleable and further neurophysiologic studies of seasonally affected horses during clinical disease and remission are warranted to investigate this. The reason for this seasonality of clinical signs and why some horses enter spontaneous long-term remission, which may last from weeks to years, is unknown. The rate at which horses enter such long-term remission seems low, with only 5% of 109 TMHS horses ceasing headshaking for more than 1 year.[2] One TMHS horse in remission has been observed to exhibit recurrence of clinical signs shortly after receiving an electric shock to the muzzle (J. Madigan, personal communication, 2011).

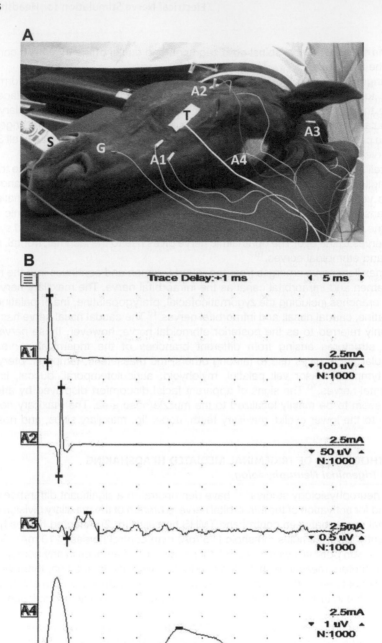

Fig. 2. Sensory nerve conduction study. (*A*) Stimulating unit (S) located in the maxillary gingival mucosa and recording electrodes (pair per site, labeled as A1, A2, A3, A4). A1, infraorbital nerve; A2, maxillary nerve; A3, spinal tract of trigeminal complex; A4, cortical somatosensory; G, ground electrode; T, temperature probe. (*B*) Sensory nerve action potentials recorded in a horse with idiopathic headshaking at areas A1, A2, A3, and A4. Note the low stimulus intensity at 2.5 milliamperes (mA); divisions: 5 milliseconds (ms) per horizontal division; variable amplitude in microvolts (μV) per vertical divisions as indicated; N, average of 1000 responses. (*From* Pickles K, Madigan J, Aleman M. Idiopathic headshaking: is it still idiopathic? Vet J. 2014 Jul;201(1):21–30; with permission.)

Cause of Trigeminal Nerve Sensitization

The cause of this aberrant trigeminal nerve activity ("sensitization") in TMHS remains obscure. A common cause of trigeminal neuropathic pain in humans occurs as a complication of shingles, the reactivation of the latent herpesvirus varicella-zoster virus. Despite the predilection of equine herpesvirus 1 for latency in the trigeminal ganglia, there was no significant difference in quantitation of equine herpesvirus-1 DNA in ganglia from control and TMHS horses,[12] suggesting a role for this virus is unlikely.

Some clinical similarities seem to exist between TMHS and HTN, a debilitating cause of facial pain in people. Unlike equine TMHS, however, patients with HTN usually have unilateral clinical signs[8] and demyelination of the ipsilateral trigeminal nerve root entry zone associated with focal compression by overlying blood vessels is frequently documented.[13,14] Such anatomy and pathology favors the ectopic generation of spontaneous nerve impulses and their ephaptic transmission to adjacent fibers, the likelihood of which is increased by the pathologic condition caused by vascular compression.[13] Neither demyelination injury[6,15,16] nor the reduced conduction velocity,[11] which would be caused by such lesions, have been found in trigeminal nerve studies of headshaking horses. HTN, like TMHS, is paroxysmal in nature and therefore some investigators argue that such clinical signs are inconsistent with compression-induced ectopic impulses at the site of injury. Spontaneous discharges arising from select neurons whose threshold for firing has been altered has been proposed as a more plausible explanation[8] and this hypothesis is compatible with the neurophysiologic studies reported in horses with TMHS.[6] TMHS may therefore be useful as an animal model for studying a naturally occurring trigeminal nerve disorder with altered threshold activity. Dorsal root ganglion cells have been shown to possess properties that (in certain circumstances) can lead to this type of spontaneous firing activity.[17] Increase in subthreshold oscillations in the resting membrane potential of a subpopulation of A neurons[18] leads to increased spike activity and subsequent cross-excitation of adjacent hyperexcitable C fibers.[19] A nociceptive signal of pain results if sufficient neurons are recruited into this spreading cluster of discharging cells.[19] Inherent cell self-quenching mechanisms are believed to cause the abrupt cessation of such signals (and thus pain). Patients with HTN with continuous ectopic discharge and unrelenting pain may have central sensitization or progressive damage to the central terminals of trigeminal afferents.[20]

Because horses with TMHS can go into spontaneous seasonal, or less frequently long-term, remission, sometimes after many years of TMHS, it seems that the aberrant trigeminal nerve activity might be reversible. Together these findings suggest functional rather than structural alterations in the trigeminal nerve in equine TMHS; however, neurophysiologic studies to investigate this hypothesis have not been performed.

It has been postulated that the photic trigger to clinical signs in some horses with TMHS is similar to the human photic sneeze[21] in which persistent photic stimulation via the optic nerve leads to a tickling sensation in the nasal mucosa.[22] The neural pathway of this phenomenon could be the result of intense light stimulation of the optic nerves causing cross-activation of the maxillary branch of the trigeminal nerve.[23] A second theory called "parasympathetic generalization," postulates that adjacently located parasympathetic branches are coactivated.[23] Similar neural pathways could be involved in causing irritating sensations and subsequent TMHS behavior in horses triggered by bright light.[21] The clinical signs of photic TMHS are identical to those of nonphotic TMHS[2,15] and therefore multiple triggers seem to activate the same end trigeminal response. Indeed, TMHS can also be triggered by sound (metal sound, clap) or eating (hard carrots, fibrous hay) and a worsening of headshaking may follow a diagnostic nasal swab or when food is in contact with the nose.[11]

Exercise is a stimulus for TMHS activity in many horses.[1,21,24] The reason for this is unclear but perhaps increased air currents over the nose result in allodynia in affected horses. Geldings consistently seem to be overrepresented (odds ratio 2.16),[2,3] although the reason for this is also puzzling. Lack of testosterone-induced negative feedback of gonadotropins was investigated as a hypothesis for this (and the seasonality of clinical signs) but was not upheld.[25] Seasonal fluctuations in pasture nutritive value, particularly improved grassland, might offer an alternative explanation for the seasonality of TMHS clinical signs, and investigation of such an association is currently ongoing.[26]

LIMITATIONS OF TREATMENT OF TRIGEMINAL MEDIATED HEADSHAKING

Treatment of TMHS is frustrating with most of the horses being *managed* (which is not always possible) rather than cured. The high failure rate of many TMHS treatments is unsurprising given that they have no effect on correcting the abnormal trigeminal neurophysiology. In addition, because the cause of the underlying trigeminal sensitization is unknown, most treatments used in TMHS are neither specific nor curative. The lack of gross pathology and the fact that some headshaking horses go into spontaneous seasonal and long-term remission suggests that the causal trigeminal nerve sensitization can be reversible. This offers hope that manipulation of the threshold activation of the trigeminal nerve could be a curative treatment for TMHS.

Validation of any new treatment is compounded by the difficulty in objective quantitative assessment of the condition and any treatment response, the phenomena of spontaneous and seasonal remission and placebo effect. A significant placebo effect has been evidenced by blinded trials of headshaking treatments using owner-assessed response to treatment.[25,27] A grading system has been proposed[28] where the severity of headshaking is graded as follows:

0/3 = no headshaking; 1/3 = headshaking at exercise but insufficiently severe as to interfere with ridden exercise; 2/3 = headshaking at exercise, of a severity sufficient to make riding impossible or dangerous; 3/3 = headshaking even at rest, in the stable and/or field.

Consensus and adoption of a standard grading system would be advantageous for comparison of future research studies.

ELECTRICAL NERVE STIMULATION

Electrical nerve stimulation is the therapeutic alteration of activity in the central, peripheral, or autonomic nervous systems by transcutaneous or implanted electrical devices. Two such therapies, percutaneous electrical nerve stimulation (PENS) and electroacupuncture, have recently been reported as successful in the management of TMHS.[28–30]

Therapeutic application of electricity dates back thousands of years to when the ancient Egyptians used electric fish for analgesia.[31] Following widespread use in the nineteenth century, the advent of modern analgesic drugs led to a wane in electrotherapy until publication of the gate control theory of pain[32] led to a resurgence of interest in neurostimulation. The principle of gate control theory is the scientific foundation underlying the mild analgesic effect derived from rubbing a painful body part. Gate control theory states that the substantia gelatinosa in the dorsal horn of the spinal cord acts as a gate control system, which modulates the synaptic transmission of nerve impulses from peripheral fibers to the central nervous system. Small nociceptive A-δ and C fibers hold the "gate" in an open position, whereas stimulation of large mechanoreceptive A-β fibers by touch, pressure, or vibration close the "gate" and inhibit pain transmission to the brain. Small nociceptive fibers have a higher activation threshold than larger mechanoreceptive fibers, such that selective low-level stimulation of mechanoreceptors can prevent or reduce pain transmission. Activation of these large A-β fibers recruits inhibitory interneurons within the substantia gelatinosa of the spinal cord that exert their inhibitory action on both large- and small-diameter fibers synapsing higher up the spinal cord. In addition, activation of the descending inhibitory pathway, which starts in the periaqueductal gray matter of the midbrain and passes through the ventral medulla into the spinal cord, occurs. Activation of this pathway results in the enhanced release of endogenous opioids[33] and alterations of many other neuroexcitatory or neuroinhibitory compounds, including serotonin, noradrenaline, gamma aminobutyric acid, acetylcholine, substance P, and adenosine.[31]

Electrical Stimulation for Treatment of Human Trigeminal Neuropathic Pain

Electrotherapy of human neuromusculoskeletal pain is currently performed using transcutaneous electrical nerve stimulation (TENS), PENS, and spinal cord stimulation (SCS). In mild to moderate pain TENS is effective, whereas PENS and SCS are useful for therapy of refractory neuropathic or ischemic pain, with PENS used for localized pain treatment.[31] The electrical devices differ in regard to the amplitude (intensity), frequency, duration, and pattern of the electrical currents.

PENS, which allows precise subcutaneous field stimulation targeted to specific areas of neuropathic pain, is a recognized treatment under National Institute for Health and Care Excellence guidelines for human sufferers of neuropathic pain in the United Kingdom.[34] It has proved effective in decreasing both subjective and objective pain scores in a randomized, double-blind, sham-controlled, crossover trial of 31 patients with chronic pain and surface hyperalgesia[35] and has been successfully used for the treatment of neuropathic trigeminal pain syndromes.[36,37] Seven out of 10 (70%) patients with postherpetic or traumatic trigeminal neuropathic pain treated with PENS of the supraorbital or infraorbital nerves reported reduction in pain of at least 50% at 24 months.[36] Similarly, 22 of 30 (73%) patients experienced more than a 50% reduction in pain following PENS stimulation of the trigeminal and/or occipital peripheral for intractable craniofacial pain.[37]

It is important to note the paucity of basic science or electrophysiologic studies demonstrating how electrical nerve stimulation has an analgesic effect. Gate control theory, whereby nociceptive information from small diameter afferents is overridden by the stimulation of large diameter fibers, is used to explain the action of high-frequency electrical stimulation.[32] It is the activation of large-diameter primary afferents from deep somatic tissues, and not cutaneous afferents, that seems to be pivotal in causing TENS analgesia.[38] TENS have been shown to gate the somatosensory transmission, both at this peripheral level and also centrally at the level of the cuneatus nucleus.[39] Low-frequency and high-frequency TENS has been shown to produce a nociceptive effect by descending inhibitory pathways, namely activation of μ- and δ-opioid receptors, respectively, in the rostral ventral medulla.[33]

There are few contraindications to electrotherapy although in humans it is advised not to use neurostimulation devices in cases with demand-type cardiac pacemakers, epilepsy, and pregnancy. To the author's knowledge, electrical nerve stimulation has not been performed on a pregnant mare to date.

Electrical Stimulation in Trigeminal Mediated Headshaking

Percutaneous electrical nerve stimulation

The recently developed, equine-specific, neurostimulation technique trademarked as EquiPENS has been used to provide stimulation of the infraorbital nerve (Video 1) in more than 130 TMHS horses, with approximately 50% successfully returning to the previous level of activity for a period of time.[28,30] As such it is the recommended treatment for horses that do not respond to simple measures such as nose nets.[28] This procedure uses an electrically conductive PENS therapy probe[a], which is conductive over its whole length attached to a neurostimulator to provide an alternating 2 and 100 Hz frequency current to the nerve. The device is voltage controlled with the current delivered varying in line with potentially varying impedances encountered (such as distance of placement from the nerve fibers) and being set by the patient's response of twitching of the facial muscles within their tolerance level for the procedure.

When neurostimulation is initiated, some horses seem to act as if surprised. Others may react quite strongly, throwing the head and snorting for the first few seconds to minutes, which seems to be eased by rubbing the nose. Horses then settle and tolerate the procedure well, even when under a low plane of sedation. Anecdotally, people undergoing PENS therapy report the procedure gives a pleasant sensation, although placement of the probe can be uncomfortable.

Complications are reported in 9% of horses following PENS therapy[30] and include slight swelling or, less frequently, a hematoma of the insertion area. Infection is a possible complication although has not been reported to date in more than 530 procedures.[30] A transient worsening of headshaking is observed in 3% of horses following PENS, which is presumed to be caused by temporary neuritis. Headshaking signs in these horses returned to baseline or less within a few days, and this temporary exacerbation does not seem to affect likelihood of successful therapy.[30] Similarly, a transient increase in pain is occasionally reported by human recipients of PENS therapy for a few hours to days or weeks following a procedure but may still go on to experience remission. There have been no reports of long-term complications following PENS treatment in humans.

The response to EquiPENS is individual and variable and a series of 3 initial treatments is required to determine if therapy has been successful.[28] It is recognized in human medicine that response to treatment for neuropathic pain varies amongst individuals, even with the same diagnosis.[40] PENS therapy of 136 horses with TMHS reported 53% of horses in remission following the initial 3 procedures.[30] Median length of remission following the third treatment has been reported as 15.5 weeks (range 0–24 weeks, n = 5)[28] and 9.5 weeks (range 2 days to 156 weeks and ongoing, n = 136).[30] Further stimulation procedures can be given as necessary at individually determined intervals as clinical signs resume or worsen.

Electroacupuncture

Electroacupuncture also provides percutaneous stimulation of the nerve and has been reported as useful in treating chronic neuropathic pain in horses and people.[41,42] The use of electroacupuncture as an additional treatment (in conjunction with face masks/nose nets) for TMHS has been reported in 6 horses.[29] In this report horses received electroacupuncture of the infraorbital nerve under light sedation. Electroacupuncture needles were connected to a stimulator unit using crocodile clips and incremental

---

[a] Manufacturer's Addresses: Algotec Research and Development, UK; The Pinnacle, Station Way, Crawley RH10 1JH, UK.

stimulation given at alternating 2 and 80 Hz frequencies until a nostril twitch was evident. Similar to EquiPENS stimulation, voltage often needed to be increased during the procedure to maintain a twitch response. The procedure was well tolerated and without any serious side effects.

Following electroacupuncture therapy, similar to PENS, response was variable and individual. All horses reduced headshaking intensity; however, the limited number of horses (n = 6) included in this study cautions against overinterpretation of this finding and the author is aware of other TMHS-affected horses that have not responded to electroacupuncture. Median remission time following the first treatment was 5.5 days (range 0–13 days, n = 6), second treatment 8.5 days (range 7–21 days, n = 6), third treatment 18 days (range 6–71 days, n = 6), fourth treatment 47.5 days (range 11 days – 25.5 weeks, n = 6), fifth treatment 13 weeks 5 days (range 5 weeks – 46 weeks n = 5), and 6th treatment 24 days (range 13–41 days n = 3).[29]

Implanted devices

There are no published studies to date using implanted devices for treatment of TMHS; however, such implants have been used successfully to manage intractable human craniofacial pain syndromes.[37,43] Following trial subcutaneous implantation over the implicated branch of the trigeminal nerve, 49% (17/35) of patients, with a variety of craniofacial pain diagnoses including 7 with trigeminal neuropathic pain, reported decreased pain. Fifteen of these patients then received permanent implants and all experienced at least temporary relief, with 11/15 reporting long-term improvement. Survival analysis predicted continued benefit in 90%, 77%, and 51% of patients at 12, 24, and 36 months postoperatively, respectively.[43] Electrode and extension wire malfunctions due to fracture or migration can occur but were not common. For those patients who experienced a reduction in analgesic effect over time, a break from stimulation seemed to allow resumption of benefit.[43] Such implants may be useful in the long-term management of TMHS in horses that respond to peripheral electrical nerve stimulation procedures such as EquiPENS or electroacupuncture and trials are warranted.

Limitations

Whilst no placebo treatment was used in the available electrical stimulation studies, the evidence suggests these treatments are useful in the management of TMHS. It can be difficult to use placebo treatment in clinical trials using privately owned horses. In addition, the difficulty in finding an appropriate placebo/sham treatment for electrical nerve stimulation studies is acknowledged in human neuromodulation studies.[44]

SUMMARY

Peripheral electrical nerve stimulation seems useful for the management of TMHS, with approximately 50% success in returning horses to their previous level of work for a variable length of time. Response to stimulation is individual and variable but is currently the safest and most effective treatment for horses that do not respond to simple physical treatments such as nose nets. Advances in the treatment of TMHS will remain limited until we fully comprehend the mechanism underlying the causal trigeminal nerve sensitization. The mechanism of action underlying any neuromodulation effect is poorly understood and further neurophysiologic research pre- and postneuromodulation, in any species, is warranted. Such studies are likely to be necessary in order to optimize electrical nerve stimulation treatment of TMHS.

SUPPLEMENTARY DATA

Supplementary data related to this article can be found online at https://doi.org/10.1016/j.cveq.2019.03.002.

REFERENCES

1. Lane JG, Mair TS. Observations on headshaking in the horse. Equine Vet J 1987; 19:331–6.
2. Madigan JE, Bell SA. Owner survey of headshaking in horses. J Am Vet Med Assoc 2001;219:334–7.
3. Mills DS, Cook S, Jones B. Reported response to treatment among 245 cases of equine headshaking. Vet Rec 2002;150:311–3.
4. Ross SE, Murray JK, Roberts VL. Prevalence of headshaking within the equine population in the UK. Equine Vet J 2018;50:73–8.
5. Williams WL. Involuntary twitching of the head relieved by trifacial neurectomy. J Comp Med Vet Arch 1897;18:426–8.
6. Aleman M, Williams DC, Brosnan RJ, et al. Sensory nerve conduction and somatosensory evoked potentials of the trigeminal nerve in horses with idiopathic headshaking. J Vet Intern Med 2013;27(6):1571–80.
7. Pickles K, Madigan J, Aleman M. Idiopathic headshaking: is it still idiopathic? Review. Vet J 2014;201(1):21–30.
8. Nurmikko TJ, Eldridge PR. Trigeminal neuralgia–pathophysiology, diagnosis and current treatment. Br J Anaesth 2001;87:117–32.
9. De Lahunta A, Glass E. Veterinary neuroanatomy and clinical neurology. 3rd edition. St Louis (MO): Saunders Elsevier; 2009.
10. Budras KD, Sack WO, Rock S, et al. Anatomy of the horse. 5th edition. Hannover (Germany): Schlutersche; 2009.
11. Aleman M, Rhodes D, Williams DC, et al. Sensory evoked potentials of the trigeminal nerve for the diagnosis of idiopathic headshaking in a horse. J Vet Intern Med 2014;28(1):250–3.
12. Aleman M, Pickles KJ, Simonek G, et al. Latent equine herpesvirus-1 in trigeminal ganglia and equine idiopathic headshaking. J Vet Intern Med 2012;26(1):192–4.
13. Love S, Coakham HB. Trigeminal neuralgia: pathology and pathogenesis. Brain 2001;124(Pt 12):2347–60.
14. Devor M, Amir R, Rappaport ZH. Pathophysiology of trigeminal neuralgia: the ignition hypothesis. Clin J Pain 2002;18(1):4–13.
15. Newton SA. The functional anatomy of the trigeminal nerve in the horse. PhD Thesis. University of Liverpool; 2001.
16. Roberts VL, Fews D, McNamara JM, et al. Trigeminal nerve root demyelination not seen in six horses diagnosed with trigeminal-mediated headshaking. Front Vet Sci 2017;4:72.
17. Amir R, Michaelis M, Devor M. Membrane potential oscillations in dorsal root ganglion neurons: role in normal excitogenesis and neuropathic pain. J Neurosci 1999;19(19):8589–96.
18. Liu CH, Wall PD, Ben-Dor E, et al. Tactile allodynia in the absence of C-fibre activation: altered firing properties of DRG neurons following spinal nerve injury. Pain 2000;85(3):503–21.
19. Amir R, Devor M. Functional cross-excitation between afferent A and C neurons in dorsal root ganglia. Neuroscience 2000;95(1):189–95.
20. Burchiel KJ, Slavin KV. On the natural history of trigeminal neuralgia. Neurosurgery 2000;46(1):152–5.

21. Madigan JE, Kortz G, Murphy C, et al. Photic headshaking in the horse: 7 cases. Equine Vet J 1995;27:306–11.
22. Whitman WW, Packer RJ. The photic sneeze reflex: literature review and discussion. Neurology 1993;43:868–71.
23. Everett HC. Sneezing in response to light. Neurology 1964;14:483–90.
24. Mair TS, Lane JG. Headshaking in horses. In Pract 1990;9:183–6.
25. Pickles KJ, Berger J, Davies R, et al. Use of a gonadotrophin-releasing hormone vaccine in headshaking horses. Vet Rec 2011;168:19.
26. Sheldon S, Aleman M, Costa L, et al. Alterations in metabolic status and headshaking behavior following intravenous administration of hypertonic solutions in horses with trigeminal-mediated headshaking. Animals 2018;8(7):102.
27. Talbot WA, Pinchbeck GL, Knottenbelt DC, et al. A randomised, blinded, crossover study to assess the efficacy of a feed supplement in alleviating the clinical signs of headshaking in 32 horses. Equine Vet J 2013;45:293–7.
28. Roberts VL, Patel NK, Tremaine WH. Neuromodulation using percutaneous electrical nerve stimulation for the management of trigeminal-mediated headshaking: a safe procedure resulting in medium-term remission in five of seven horses. Equine Vet J 2016;48:201–4.
29. Devereux S. Electroacupuncture as an additional treatment for headshaking in six horses. Equine Vet Educ 2017. https://doi.org/10.1111/eve.12776.
30. Roberts VLH, Bailey M, Carslake HB, et al. Safety and efficacy of equipens neuromodulation for the management of trigeminal-mediated headshaking in 168 horses. Equine Vet J, in press.
31. Heidland A, Fazeli G, Klassen A, et al. Neuromuscular electrostimulation techniques: historical aspects and current possibilities in treatment of pain and muscle wasting. Clin Nephrol 2013;79(Suppl. 1):S12–23.
32. Melzack R, Wall PD. Pain mechanisms: a new theory. Science 1965;150:971–9. https://doi.org/10.1126/science.150.3699.971.
33. Kalra A, Urban MO, Sluka KA. Blockade of opioid receptors in rostral ventral medulla prevents antihyperalgesia produced by transcutaneous electrical nerve stimulation (TENS). J Pharmacol Exp Ther 2001;298(1):257–63.
34. UK Department of Health. National Institute for health and care excellence guidelines. 2013. Available at: http://guidance.nice.org.uk/IPG450. Accessed April 4, 2018.
35. Raphael JH, Raheem TA, Southall JL, et al. Randomized double-blind sham-controlled crossover study of short-term effect of percutaneous electrical nerve stimulation in neuropathic pain. Pain Med 2011;12(10):1515–22.
36. Johnson MD, Burchiel KJ. Peripheral stimulation for treatment of trigeminal postherpetic neuralgia and trigeminal posttraumatic neuropathic pain: a pilot study. Neurosurgery 2004;55:135–42.
37. Slavin KV, Colpan ME, Munawar N, et al. Trigeminal and occipital peripheral nerve stimulation for craniofacial pain: a single-institution experience and review of the literature. Neurosurg Focus 2006;21:E6.
38. Radhakrishnan R, Sluka KA. Deep tissue afferents, but not cutaneous afferents, mediate transcutaneous electrical nerve stimulation–induced antihyperalgesia. J Pain 2005;6(10):673–80.
39. Nardone A, Schieppati M. Influences of transcutaneous electrical stimulation of cutaneous and mixed nerves on subcortical and cortical somatosensory evoked potentials. Electroencephalogr Clin Neurophysiol 1989;74:24–35.

40. Neuropathic pain in adults: pharmacological management in nonspecialist settings Clinical guideline [CG173]. 2013. Available at: https://www.nice.org.uk/guidance/cg173/chapter/1-Recommendations. Accessed April 4, 2018.

41. Xie H, Colahan P, Ott EA. Evaluation of electroacupuncture treatment of horses with signs of chronic thoracolumbar pain. J Am Vet Med Assoc 2005;227:281–6.

42. White PF, Li S, Chiu JW. Electroanalgesia: its role in acute and chronic pain management. Anesth Analg 2001;92:505–13.

43. Ellis JA, Mejia Munne JC, Winfree CJ. Trigeminal branch stimulation for the treatment of intractable craniofacial pain. J Neurosurg 2015;123:283–8.

44. Gybels J, Erdine S, Maeyaert J, et al. Neuromodulation of pain: a consensus statement prepared in Brussels 16–18 January 1998 by the following task force of the European Federation of IASP Chapters (EFIC). Eur J Pain 1998;2:203–9.

Is There Still a Place for Lidocaine in the (Postoperative) Management of Colics?

David E. Freeman, MVB, PhD

KEYWORDS

- Lidocaine • Colic • Horse • Postoperative reflux • Postoperative ileus
- Inflammation

KEY POINTS

- Intravenous lidocaine infusion has been widely used to prevent or treat postoperative ileus after surgery for colic in horses.
- Clinical studies support this approach, but flaws in these studies, contradictory findings from others, and the nature of the disease have raised concerns about the efficacy of lidocaine.
- Because of cost and questions about efficacy, a well-designed clinical trial is required to support continued lidocaine use.
- The analgesic properties of lidocaine as part of a multimodal strategy should be considered in select cases with postoperative colic.

INTRODUCTION

"Lidocaine has categorically been shown to have a positive effect on the small intestinal motility. It reduces ileus and acts as an anti-inflammatory, though we are not sure why. Inflammatory cells are involved with keeping the bowel from moving correctly."[1] This statement summarizes the role of lidocaine in managing horses after small intestinal surgery[1] and represents an opinion widely embraced by many equine surgeons over the last 2 decades. However, during that time, little evidence has accrued to support the role of lidocaine as a prokinetic drug or an antiinflammatory agent, although another potential role relevant to colic surgery might have emerged.

Disclosure Statement: The authors have no relationship with a commercial company that has a direct financial interest in subject matter or materials discussed in article or with a company making a competing product.

Equine Surgery, University of Florida, College of Veterinary Medicine, Large Animal Clinical Sciences, PO Box 100136, Gainesville, FL 32610, USA

E-mail address: freemand@ufl.edu

POSTOPERATIVE ILEUS

Postoperative ileus (POI) is defined as the failure of gastrointestinal motility to recover after colic surgery, is a common complication after small intestinal surgery in horses, and is the disease targeted by lidocaine.[2] Its importance arises through welfare concerns, prolonged hospitalization, increased costs of treatment, and reduced postoperative survival.[3] Postoperative reflux (POR) is considered more appropriate terminology than POI because it includes all causes of reflux (**Fig. 1**), including those that are purely physical (eg, anastomotic stricture).[3] For the remainder of this discussion, POI is used to designate the functional disease targeted by lidocaine as treatment or prevention, and POR is used to denote the major clinical manifestation of POI and other causes of reflux.[3]

Evidence that intravenous (IV) lidocaine can shorten the duration of POI in the human colon after abdominal surgery[4] prompted its widespread use for the same purpose after colic surgery in horses.[5–9] Its benefits in human patients with POI have been attributed to (1) reducing circulating catecholamines by inhibition of the sympathoadrenal response, (2) suppressing activity in the primary afferent neurons involved in reflex inhibition of intestinal motility, (3) stimulating smooth muscle directly, and (4) decreasing inflammation in the bowel wall through the inhibition of prostaglandin synthesis, the inhibition of granulocyte migration, and the release of lysosomal enzymes and free radicals.[4]

One of the earliest reports of using IV lidocaine in horses demonstrated that a loading dose of lidocaine followed by a continuous rate infusion (CRI) decreased halothane minimum alveolar concentration (MAC) in a dose-dependent fashion.[10] This approach to reducing the cardiovascular depressant effects of inhalants in anesthetized horses seems to be widely adopted[11] and even credited in 1 study as a possible means of preventing POI.[12] A survey of Diplomates of the American College of Veterinary Surgeons published in 2004 revealed that lidocaine CRI was the most commonly used prokinetic agent in horses after colic surgery (76% of respondents).[7] In recent surveys of European and American specialists that treat colic, IV lidocaine was used in 79% of all POI cases in Europe[8] and in 69% of such cases in the United

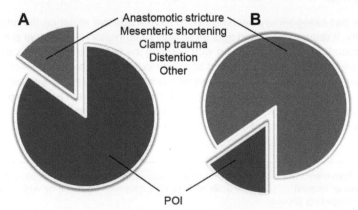

Fig. 1. Pie charts to demonstrate that POI could be one of many factors responsible for POR after small intestinal surgery, with most of the others grouped as physical causes of obstruction (anastomotic stricture, etc). The relative weighting of these factors is unknown in any individual horse with POR, but scenario A would assign POI the major role and the only opportunity for lidocaine to be effective. Repeat celiotomy could be highly effective in scenario B.

States.[9] In the same studies, 67% of European specialists used lidocaine postoperatively to prevent POI, compared with 57% in the American-based study.[8,9]

The recommended protocol for treating or preventing POI in horses with lidocaine is an initial loading dose of 1.3 mg/kg IV infused over 15 minutes, followed by 0.05 mg/kg/min in saline or lactated Ringer's solution over 24 hours.[6,13] This dose produces a serum concentration of 1 to 2 μg/mL, with 0.98 μg/mL considered the minimum therapeutic concentration.[6,13] Serum lidocaine concentrations can reach peak values during the loading infusion in awake and anesthetized horses.[14] By 3 hours after the infusion starts, horses can have a decrease in heart rate and diminished signs of existing lameness.[6] However, a significant effect on heart rate was not evident in another study, even at potentially toxic doses.[15]

METABOLISM AND PHARMACOKINETICS OF LIDOCAINE

Lidocaine IV is largely metabolized in the liver to yield increasing serum concentrations of 2 metabolites, monoethylglycinexylidide and glycinexylidide, with unknown roles in lidocaine-induced responses in horses.[5,16] Despite the substantial accumulation of these metabolites during lidocaine CRI, their concentrations and those of lidocaine return to baseline rapidly after infusion ends in healthy horses.[16] Lidocaine clearance in fed horses is approximately twice that in horses denied food, presumably because of superior hepatic blood flow in the fed state.[17]

In healthy awake horses, serum lidocaine concentrations were significantly less than in healthy anesthetized horses during loading and maintenance infusion periods in 1 study, possibly because of a decrease in cardiac output and hepatic blood flow during anesthesia.[14] These differences were not associated with adverse cardiopulmonary responses or behavioral evidence of toxicosis.[14] In a study on postoperative colic patients, lidocaine and both glycinexylidide and monoethylglycinexylidide seemed to accumulate in blood over time,[18] possibly because hepatic blood flow was reduced through hemodynamic alterations from systemic inflammation[16] and endotoxic shock.[19] This finding differs from the results of a study on lidocaine disposition in horses under anesthesia for colic surgery, in which the lidocaine concentration was lower and distribution and total body clearance values were higher than expected[20] and comparable with those recorded in healthy anesthetized horses.[14] Based on these results, horses with gastrointestinal lesions requiring surgery do not seem to require a modification of the lidocaine dose.[20]

Lidocaine is moderately protein bound in equine plasma,[21] largely to α_1-acid glycoprotein,[22] and loss of this and possibly other proteins in horses with colic could increase the plasma concentrations of lidocaine and metabolites to unsafe levels. In 1 study, the in vitro protein binding of lidocaine in equine plasma at 2 μg/mL was decreased from 53% to 29% or less when ceftiofur was given alone or combined with flunixin meglumine (FM).[21] These findings suggested that FM, which is a highly protein-bound drug, could displace lidocaine from protein and increase its unbound fraction and risk of toxicity.[21] In an in vivo study of healthy horses, the concurrent administration of lidocaine and FM did not seem to affect plasma concentration of each drug, but this study did not resolve the effects of protein binding.[23]

TOXICITY OF LIDOCAINE

Signs of toxicity in the awake horse, such as muscle fasciculations, anxiety, incoordination, ataxia, alterations in visual function, and collapse, are mediated through central nervous system effects.[15] Sudden collapse can be especially devastating in the horse after colic surgery because it can lead to some degree of dehiscence of the ventral midline incision. Altered visual function is evident as intermittent eye blinking, anxiety, and close inspection of nearby objects.[15] Loss of consciousness, seizures, and respiratory arrest can follow severe overdosing.[24]

Lidocaine has a narrow therapeutic index so that the upper end of the effective dose closely approaches the dose at which adverse responses can develop.[24] For example, toxic effects can become evident in the 1.9 to 4.5 μg/mL range, which puts the toxic threshold in the horse at 2 to 3 times the target therapeutic level used to treat POI.[15] In a study that examined the responses of healthy horses to a slightly increased loading dose and 6 times the CRI dose, muscle fasciculations were observed at mean serum concentrations of 3.24 μg/mL.[15] In this study, clinically significant cardiovascular effects did not seem to develop in horses with serum lidocaine concentrations that induced signs of toxicity in the nervous and/or musculoskeletal systems.[15] Hypovolemia, hypoproteinemia, or both could be pronounced in horses with severe gastrointestinal disease and could lead to higher concentrations of free lidocaine in plasma than in normal horses, thereby increasing the risk of toxicity at recommended doses by body weight.

Because of rapid hepatic metabolism of lidocaine and the short half-lives of its metabolites,[16] the cessation of therapy or a reduction of the infusion rate should be instituted as soon as muscle fasciculations or other toxic responses are evident.[6,13,24] A lidocaine CRI used for balanced anesthesia should cease at least 30 minutes before the end of anesthesia to prevent the exacerbation of ataxia and incoordination in the recovery stall.[11] If seizures or excitement develop, general anesthesia might be required, but diazepam should not be used because of the risk of incoordination and delirium.[24] Other possible side effects are delayed detection of pain from laminitis[6] and an increased risk of incisional infection.[25]

MECHANISM OF ACTION OF LIDOCAINE: PROKINETIC EFFECTS

Despite the widespread use of lidocaine as a prokinetic agent,[7–9] it does not seem to have a prokinetic effect, at least in the jejunum of healthy horses after surgery to implant the electrodes used to assess motility.[26] Also, a lidocaine infusion at recommended doses can either delay[27] or have no effect on intestinal transit in healthy awake horses.[28] In an in vitro study with smooth muscle strips from healthy equine stomach and intestine, lidocaine increased the contractile activity of the proximal portion of the duodenum, but did not affect the pyloric antrum or middle portion of the jejunum.[29] However, these findings might not be relevant to the same segments in horses with inflamed intestine, in which inhibitory reflexes could dominate motility patterns.[29] Although lidocaine can improve smooth muscle contractility in vitro in equine jejunum after ischemia/reperfusion injury in vivo,[30] the concentrations required to achieve this response far exceed safe plasma concentrations. Lidocaine can block the Na^+ current through channels in jejunal circular muscle that can contribute to slow wave generation,[31] an effect that would not be expected to enhance motility. Also, coordinated pressure peaks in the equine colon can be markedly diminished by slow topical application of lidocaine around the colic arteries, and this response, if induced by systemic lidocaine, could interfere with normal colonic motility.[32]

MECHANISM OF ACTION OF LIDOCAINE: ANTIINFLAMMATORY EFFECTS

The putative antiinflammatory effects of lidocaine could be of benefit to horses with POI because of the proposed role of inflammation in the pathogenesis of this complication.[33] The current hypothesis for development of POI proposes an early neurogenic and a later inflammatory response to gastrointestinal surgery,[33] which has recently been incorporated into 4 phases, as follows[34]:

- An early neurogenic phase caused by surgery and mediated through the activation of mesenteric and splanchnic afferent nerves, eventually leading to impaired motility through nitrergic and adrenergic effects.[34] This phase usually ends with termination of surgery.[34]
- An early phase of inhibited smooth muscle function (lasting until 6 hours after intestinal manipulation) mediated in part by innate cytokines released, most likely by resident macrophages. This inflammatory phase is probably triggered by intestinal manipulation and involves interaction between the immune system, the autonomic nervous system, and gastrointestinal smooth muscle.[34]
- A second phase of smooth muscle inhibition starts after approximately 6 hours, is temporally associated with the influx of inflammatory cells, and lasts until 24 hours after intestinal manipulation.
- The final phase involves alterations in enteric neurotransmission and cholinergic activity that can persist after the recovery of gastrointestinal transit.[34]

Lidocaine can inhibit neutrophil adhesion, migration, phagocytosis, and free radical production,[35] can downregulate nuclear factor-$\kappa\beta$ signaling,[36] and inhibit tumor necrosis factor-α, IL-2, and IL-8 production during inflammation induced by ischemia.[36–38] Despite these potential beneficial effects in other animals, there is little evidence that lidocaine might actually produce an antiinflammatory effect in any organ in horses. In an in vitro study on equine neutrophils, lidocaine did not inhibit neutrophil migration or adhesion at therapeutic concentrations, and it actually increased migration and adhesion at potentially toxic concentrations.[39] It also failed to reduce the expression of proinflammatory genes in lipopolysaccharide-stimulated equine monocytes.[40] Despite its ability to decrease inflammation and improve lung function in human asthmatic patients, lidocaine seemed to increase total cell numbers and the percentage of neutrophils in the bronchoalveolar lavage fluid from horses with recurrent airway obstruction.[41] In the black walnut model of laminitis, lidocaine increased laminar E-selectin messenger RNA concentrations and did not inhibit inflammatory events in either the laminae or the skin.[42] Systemic lidocaine at levels used to manage laminitic pain failed to change surface expression of CD13 and CD18 markers of neutrophil activation in horses that received black walnut extract.[43] In a study in which horses received intraperitoneal endotoxin, the clinical score and tumor necrosis factor-α activity were significantly lower in those treated with lidocaine than in a saline-treated group.[44] However, lidocaine had no effect on the polymorphonuclear neutrophils (PMN) cell count, fibrinogen, and total protein in peritoneal fluid and did not change IL-6 production.[44]

Lidocaine combined with FM ameliorated the inflammation (based on mucosal neutrophil counts) associated with FM alone at 18 hours of reperfusion after ischemia in adult horses.[45] In the same study, lidocaine administered IV during reperfusion reduced plasma prostaglandin E_2 metabolite concentration and mucosal cyclooxygenase-2 expression in ischemia-injured jejunum.[45] In more recent studies on transmural inflammation induced by ischemia/reperfusion or manipulation in equine jejunum and ischemia/reperfusion in equine colon, lidocaine did not blunt the inflammatory response in any intestinal layer.[46] Lidocaine did decrease cyclooxygenase-2 expression in circular muscle and through all layers combined in manipulated jejunum, but the response was not consistent and was absent in postischemic segments.[46] In another ischemia/reperfusion model in horse jejunum, moderate to severe pulmonary inflammation developed as a remote organ response, with the recruitment of neutrophils and inflammatory molecules.[47] Lidocaine decreased the pulmonary neutrophil response, but without affecting other markers of inflammation and was associated with an increase in pulmonary macrophages.[47] These findings led to an inconclusive assessment of the antiinflammatory benefits of lidocaine in this model.[47] In a study of remote organ responses in equine liver, lung, and kidney to intestinal injury induced by ischemia/reperfusion and jejunal manipulation, lidocaine did not blunt inflammation in these organs.[48]

MECHANISM OF ACTION OF LIDOCAINE: VISCERAL ANALGESIA

Perioperative lidocaine provides considerable pain relief for human patients undergoing abdominal surgery, sufficient to decrease postoperative opioid requirements and thereby reduce the adverse effects of these drugs on intestinal function.[49] This visceral pain relief could be partly explained by the inhibition of spinal neuronal populations excited by intestinal distension.[50] Anecdotal evidence has emerged that lidocaine also provides visceral analgesia in horses, although the available scientific information is inconclusive. One study had technical limitations that prevented the recording of lidocaine effects on visceral pain in a statistically meaningful number of horses.[51] However, in a study on recovery from ischemia/reperfusion in equine jejunum, lidocaine combined with FM had superior pain scores than lidocaine or FM alone.[52] This apparent benefit of lidocaine as a component of a multimodal approach to analgesia could be useful in managing horses with postoperative colic after small intestinal surgery or large colon resection. Pain relief could be of benefit in managing POI, because pain could play a contributory role in the early and late phases of this complication by mediating a sympathetic efferent response that decreases intestinal motility.[53]

MECHANISM OF ACTION OF LIDOCAINE: MISCELLANEOUS

The perceived clinical benefits of lidocaine in horses after colic surgery could also be attributed to miscellaneous effects mediated through specific peripheral and central Na^+ channels.[24] Lidocaine can prevent fluid secretion into the small intestinal lumen and decrease edema formation in the intestinal wall in rats,[54–56] effects that could benefit horses with POR or duodenitis proximal jejunitis. Lidocaine could ameliorate the increased lipopolysaccharide permeability associated with the apparent adverse effects of FM on recovery of the mucosal barrier in equine jejunal mucosa.[52] By decreasing mucosal injury and improving intestinal repair in equine jejunum and the right dorsal colon after ischemia, lidocaine could decrease the output of neutrophil chemoattractants from damaged tissue at these sites.[40]

EFFICACY OF LIDOCAINE IN THE PREVENTION AND TREATMENT OF POSTOPERATIVE ILEUS

Although POI is the postoperative complication at which lidocaine is directed for treatment and prevention, this is a difficult complication to study, for the following reasons.

- Reflux through a nasogastric tube or POR is the hallmark of POI, but could also be caused by a physical obstruction, without any indicators that would distinguish between the 2 causes.[2,3] Therefore, POI might be part of a multifactorial disease, and with an unknown overall contribution to severity of that disease (see **Fig. 1**).[3] Without surgery or necropsy, POI is only a presumptive diagnosis in any horse with POR.[3]
- In horses subjected to repeat celiotomy in a recent study, 81% responded with a complete cessation of POR after the second surgery, despite a second bout of

surgical manipulation and associated inflammation.[57] These findings demonstrate 2 ways in which lidocaine could fail in management of POR: first, the target abnormality for lidocaine (inflammation) is not the predominant cause of POR, and second, the predominant cause of POR in this study[57] and probably others (physical obstruction) is not affected by lidocaine (see **Fig. 1**).

- In 1 prospective study,[13] 19 horses with POR were excluded because reflux ceased at the onset of lidocaine/saline infusion, raising the possibility that resolution of POR during these infusions could also be a spontaneous event.[58] This is a complicating issue in studying the treatment of any disease capable of spontaneous resolution.[58]
- Cessation of POR with medical treatment could also be caused by spontaneous resolution of a physical obstruction or adaptation to it over time (eg, adhesion, anastomotic stricture), and not to a favorable response of POI to treatment.

The results of 4 studies that examined the effects of a lidocaine CRI in horses after colic surgery supported its role for treatment or prevention of POI[12,13,59,60] **(Table 1)**. However, these studies have flaws in their design or interpretation that diminish their impact, largely through insufficient study power (see **Table 1**). Also grouping large and small intestinal obstructions together and including duodenitis proximal jejunitis, presumably to increase the power of data analysis, could introduce different elements of pathogenesis and hence different responses to treatment. One retrospective study found that lidocaine CRI had no effect on the prevalence of POR, total reflux volume, duration of reflux, or survival after surgery for small intestinal colics in horses.[61] In this study, the cohorts for comparison were grouped by period of hospital admission, an early period when lidocaine was not used and later when it was. Therefore, assignment to treatment group was not random and also horses at risk of POR or that developed POR were more likely to be treated with lidocaine in this study.[61] Despite limitations related to the retrospective, nonrandomized nature of this study, the 2 groups were similar for most variables measured.[61] As with any retrospective, nonblinded studies, the latter study and possibly others (see **Table 1**) that have investigated lidocaine[12,60] have important potential biases that could render them unsuitable for meta-analysis.[62]

Important information about the benefit of any drug can be gained through studies that examine prevalence of the target disease when the drug in question is not used. Four interrelated studies demonstrated that low rates of POR were achieved after small intestinal surgery in horses without lidocaine, despite use of very inclusive criteria for POR.[63–66] These studies also used an approach to small intestinal surgery that gave every horse with a financial option for surgery a chance, regardless of disease severity, type of anastomosis indicated, and need for repeat celiotomy.[64–66] In one of these studies, no horse had POR after jejunojejunostomy.[65] By contrast, POR rates of 63% were recorded in a similar study, but with postoperative lidocaine infusion.[67] These findings underscore the importance of other factors on outcome in clinical trials on colic surgery.[68]

CONCERNS ABOUT USE OF LIDOCAINE

In the absence of an established effect of lidocaine as a prokinetic drug through direct or indirect mechanisms, the negative implications of its use need to be considered. The risk and nature of toxic effects would be acceptable, especially if the benefits were more favorable. The cost of treatment with lidocaine can be high because of the volumes required for the bolus infusion and a 24-hour (or longer) CRI, and for use of a fluid pump to ensure a safe rate of delivery. The cost of colic surgery probably

Table 1
Four studies that yielded favorable responses to lidocaine as treatment or as a prophylactic measure against POI

	Brianceau et al,[59] 2002, JVIM	Cohen et al,[12] 2004, JAVMA	Malone et al,[13] 2006, Vet Surg	Torfs et al,[60] 2009, JVIM
Study type	Randomized controlled trial, blinded, 13 lidocaine-treated horses and 15 saline controls with surgery for intestinal disease	Prospective case-control study on risk factors for POI in 2 hospital populations	Randomized controlled trial, double-blinded, prospective study, multicenter, with 17 treated horses and 15 controls	Retrospective cross-sectional study 126 horses (67% strangulating, 33% nonstrangulating lesions) 44% of all horses had SI resection and anastomosis
Timing	Intraoperative administration and continued for 24 hours postoperatively; loading dose followed by CRI	Intraoperative administration of lidocaine (details of doses not given)	24-hour CRI after lidocaine bolus Horses included if a presumptive diagnosis of duodenitis proximal jejunitis or POI with gastric reflux; no motility agents permitted in the 24 hours before and 36 hours after treatment	Horses were started on lidocaine CRI after administration of loading bolus during anesthesia (all but 11 horses). Prophylactic lidocaine after anesthesia (bolus and CRI) Horses received nonrandomized treatment with prokinetic drugs (88%); some were administered prophylactically and others once POR had developed Many horses received concurrent multiple prokinetic drugs
Results	Lidocaine CRI significantly reduced jejunal cross-section and peritoneal fluid accumulation on ultrasound examination. No effect on gastrointestinal sounds, time to passage of feces, number of defecations in first 24 hours, gastric reflux, duodenal or jejunal wall thickness, maximum duodenal or jejunal diameter or cross-sectional area, small-intestinal contractions per minute, rate of complications, or outcome.	POI developed in 47 of 251 horses Marginal association with reduced likelihood of POI with lidocaine; the inclusion of the variable intraoperative lidocaine improved model fit and hence this variable was retained	65% of treated horses with POI stopped refluxing within 30 hours, compared with 27% in the placebo group ($P = .04$) Reduced hourly volume of reflux and decreased duration of hospitalization in the lidocaine compared with the placebo group No effect on survival between lidocaine and placebo groups	Decreased risk of POI with lidocaine (51% compared with 21%) Survival odds: 3.33 times higher with lidocaine 34% survival from POI

| Flaws | Low study power and few had small intestinal lesions (n = 4 in lidocaine, n = 4 in saline group) Low prevalence of gastric reflux (n = 1 in lidocaine and n = 1 in saline group) so unable to investigate effect of lidocaine on POI | Lidocaine administration biased toward 1 hospital population Not randomized and unknown if preferential administration to horses more likely to develop POI | Lidocaine or placebo was only started after the onset of postoperative reflux and therefore cannot be used to assess its use to prevent POR No selection criteria described Duodenitis proximal jejunitis horses grouped with POI Included types of colic not typically associated with POI (colon diseases, impactions, duodenitis proximal jejunitis) Little overlap in study periods between hospitals Small numbers in different categories – low power | No apparent randomization of treatment Potential biases, for example, assignment to lidocaine group All but 11 horses received lidocaine under anesthesia Only 35 horses in the nonlidocaine group and unclear if these horses received other prokinetic drugs No apparent blinding 79% of control horses received lidocaine under anesthesia Lidocaine combined with prokinetic drugs – low power in treatment categories and role of other drugs unknown Small numbers in different categories – low power |

leads to more deaths among the general equine population with this devastating disease than disease-related factors, so that the cost to benefit ratio for lidocaine might not be acceptable. The low rate of POR recorded in studies that did not use lidocaine[63–66] suggests that POR might be a complicated disease in horses, with mixed elements of physical and functional causes that we need to unravel.

SUMMARY

The effectiveness of lidocaine as a prokinetic drug (whether through direct or indirect mechanisms) is controversial. The favorable results in horses with small intestinal disease not treated with lidocaine challenge any notions about the need to use it. However, selective use, as opposed to the current almost routine use, should be considered for horses in which a multimodal form of analgesia is required, especially combined with FM.[52] In such cases, lidocaine would offer the benefit over other analgesic drugs of having little if any adverse effect on intestinal motility. Suitable candidates would include horses that are painful after large colon resection or any gastrointestinal surgery, but with a level of pain that is manageable on the humane level. Care must be taken in postoperative small intestinal cases to ensure that signs of pain indicative of the need for repeat celiotomy are not masked by overzealous use of any analgesic drugs. The current routine use of lidocaine as a prophylactic measure against POR after small intestinal surgery is not justified, unless a large, well-designed multicenter, blinded, randomized, controlled trial proves otherwise. That POR would respond to treatment with one drug seems unrealistic, based on consideration of possible causes of this disease.

REFERENCES

1. Blikslager AT, Tiffany LM. Lots of theories, few answers on colic. Veterinary Practice News 2011;41–2. Available at: https://www.veterinarypracticenews.com/lots-of-theories-few-answers-on-colic/.
2. Merritt AM, Blikslager AT. Post operative ileus: to be or not to be? Equine Vet J 2008;40(4):295–6.
3. Freeman DE. Post-operative reflux – a surgeon's perspective. Equine Vet Educ 2018;30:671–80.
4. Rimback G, Cassuto J, Tollesson PO. Treatment of postoperative paralytic ileus by intravenous lidocaine infusion. Anesth Analg 1990;70:414–9.
5. Cook VL, Blikslager AT. Use of systemically administered lidocaine in horses with gastrointestinal tract disease. J Am Vet Med Assoc 2008;232:1144–8.
6. Malone ED, Turner TA, Wilson JH. Intravenous lidocaine for the treatment of ileus in the horse. In Proceedings of 5th Equine Colic Research Symposium, University of Georgia, Athens, 1994, p. 39.
7. Van Hoogmoed LM, Nieto JE, Snyder JR, et al. Survey of prokinetic use in horses with gastrointestinal injury. Vet Surg 2004;33:279–85.
8. Lefebvre D, Pirie RS, Handel IG, et al. Clinical features and management of equine post operative ileus: survey of diplomates of the European Colleges of Equine Internal Medicine (ECEIM) and Veterinary Surgeons (ECVS). Equine Vet J 2016;48:182–7.
9. Lefebvre D, Hudson NPH, Elce YA, et al. Clinical features and management of equine post operative ileus (POI): survey of diplomates of the American Colleges of Veterinary Internal Medicine (ACVIM), Veterinary Surgeons (ACVS) and Veterinary Emergency and Critical Care (ACVECC). Equine Vet J 2016;48:714–9.

10. Doherty TJ, Frazier DL. Effect of intravenous lidocaine on halothane minimum alveolar concentration in ponies. Equine Vet J 1998;30(4):300–3.

11. Valverde A. Balanced anesthesia and constant-rate infusions in horses. Vet Clin North Am Equine Pract 2013;29:89–122.

12. Cohen ND, Lester GD, Sanchez LC, et al. Evaluation of risk factors associated with development of postoperative ileus in horses. J Am Vet Med Assoc 2004; 225:1070–8.

13. Malone E, Ensink J, Turner T, et al. Intravenous continuous infusion of lidocaine for treatment of equine ileus. Vet Surg 2006;35:60–6.

14. Feary DJ, Mama KR, Wagner AE, et al. Influence of general anesthesia on pharmacokinetics of intravenous lidocaine infusion in horses. Am J Vet Res 2005;66: 574–80.

15. Meyer GA, Lin HC, Hanson RR, et al. Effects of intravenous lidocaine overdose on cardiac electrical activity and blood pressure in the horse. Equine Vet J 2001;33: 434–7.

16. Dickey EJ, McKenzie HC III, Brown JA, et al. Serum concentrations of lidocaine and its metabolites after prolonged infusion in healthy horses. Equine Vet J 2008; 40:348–52.

17. Engelking LR, Blyden GT, Lofsledt J, et al. Pharmacokinetics of antipyrine, acetaminophen and lidocaine in fed and fasted horses. J Vet Pharmacol Ther 1987; 10:73–82.

18. de Solís CN, McKenzie HC III. Serum concentrations of lidocaine and its metabolites MEGX and GX during and after prolonged intravenous infusion of lidocaine in horses after colic surgery. J Equine Vet Sci 2007;27:398–404.

19. McKindley DS, Boulet J, Sachdeva K, et al. Endotoxic shock alters the pharmacokinetics of lidocaine and monoethylglycinexylidide. Shock 2002;17:199–204.

20. Feary DJ, Mama KR, Thomasy SM, et al. Influence of gastrointestinal tract disease on pharmacokinetics of lidocaine after intravenous infusion in anesthetized horses. Am J Vet Res 2006;67:317–22.

21. Milligan M, Kukanich B, Beard W, et al. The disposition of lidocaine during a 12-hour intravenous infusion to postoperative horses. J Vet Pharmacol Ther 2006;29: 495–9.

22. Routledge PA, Barchowsky A, Bjornsson TD, et al. Lidocaine plasma protein binding. Clin Pharmacol Ther 1980;27:347–51.

23. Waxman SJ, Kukanich B, Milligan M, et al. Pharmacokinetics of concurrently administered intravenous lidocaine and flunixin in healthy horses. J Vet Pharmacol Ther 2011;35:413–6.

24. Vigani A, Garcia-Pereira FL. Anesthesia and analgesia for standing equine surgery. Vet Clin Equine 2014;30:1–17.

25. Stephen JO, Corley KT, Johnston JK, et al. Factors associated with mortality and morbidity in small intestinal volvulus in horses. Vet Surg 2004;33:40–348.

26. Milligan M, Beard W, Kukanich B, et al. The effect of lidocaine on postoperative jejunal motility in normal horses. Vet Surg 2007;36:214–20.

27. Rusiecki KE, Nieto JE, Puchalski SM, et al. Evaluation of continuous infusion of lidocaine on gastrointestinal tract function in normal horses. Vet Surg 2008;37: 564–70.

28. Elfenbein JR, Robertson SA, MacKay RJ, et al. Systemic and anti -nociceptive effects of prolonged lidocaine, ketamine, and butorphanol infusions alone and in combination in healthy horses. BMC Vet Res 2014;10(Suppl 1):S6.

29. Nieto JE, Rakestraw PC, Snyder JR, et al. In vitro effects of erythromycin, lidocaine, and metoclopramide on smooth muscle from the pyloric antrum, proximal

portion of the duodenum, and middle portion of the jejunum of horses. Am J Vet Res 2000;61:413–9.

30. Guschlbauer M, Hoppe S, Geburek F, et al. In vitro effects of lidocaine on the contractility of equine jejunal smooth muscle challenged by ischaemia-reperfusion injury. Equine Vet J 2010;42:53–8.

31. Holm AN, Rich A, Miller SM, et al. Sodium current in human jejunal circular smooth muscle cells. Gastroenterology 2002;122:178–87.

32. Sellers AF, Lowe JE, Brondhum J. Motor events in equine large colon. Am J Physiol 1979;237:E457–64.

33. Bauer AJ, Schwarz NT, Moore BA, et al. Ileus in critical illness: mechanisms and management. Curr Opin Crit Care 2002;8:152–7.

34. Farro G, Gomez-Pinilla PJ, Di Giovangiulio M, et al. Smooth muscle and neural dysfunction contribute to different phases of murine postoperative ileus. Neurogastroenterol Motil 2016;28:934–47.

35. Azuma Y, Shinohara M, Wang PL, et al. Comparison of inhibitory effects of local anesthetics on immune functions of neutrophils. Int J Immunopharmacol 2000;22:789–96.

36. Lahat A, Horin SB, Lang A, et al. Lidocaine down-regulates nuclear factor-κβ signalling, and inhibits cytokine production and T cell proliferation. Clin Exp Immunol 2008;152:320–7.

37. Lan W, Harmon D, Wang JH, et al. The effect of lidocaine on neutrophil CD11b/CD18 and endothelial ICAM-1 expression and IL-1β concentrations induced by hypoxia-reoxygenation. Eur J Anaesthesiol 2004;21:967–72.

38. Lang A, Horin SB, Picard O, et al. Lidocaine inhibits epithelial chemokine secretion via inhibition of nuclear factor κβ activation. Immunobiology 2010;215:304–13.

39. Cook VL, Neuder LE, Blikslager AT, et al. The effect of lidocaine on in vitro adhesion and migration of equine neutrophils. Vet Immunol Immunopathol 2009;129:137–42.

40. Cook VL. Lidocaine: we all use it – now we know why. In: Proceedings of the International Veterinary Emergency and Critical Care Symposium 2012, San Antonio, Texas. Available at: https://www.vin.com/Members/login/login.aspx?ReturnUrl=/members/proceedings/Proceedings.plx?CID=IVECCS2012&Category=&PID=85257&O=VIN. Accessed April 9, 2019.

41. Wilson ME, Berney C, Behan A, et al. Lidocaine does not prevent neutrophil influx or attenuate lung function in heaves-affected horses. J Vet Intern Med 2012;26:1427–32.

42. Williams JM, Lin YJ, Loftus JP, et al. Effect of intravenous lidocaine administration on laminar inflammation in the black walnut extract model of laminitis. Equine Vet J 2010;42:261–9.

43. Loftus JP, Williams JM, Belknap JK, et al. In vivo priming and ex vivo activation of equine neutrophils in black walnut extract-induced equine laminitis is not attenuated by systemic lidocaine administration. Vet Immunol Immunopathol 2010;138:60–9.

44. Peiro JR, Barnabe PA, Cadioli FA, et al. Effects of lidocaine infusion during experimental endotoxemia in horses. J Vet Intern Med 2010;24:940–8.

45. Cook VL, Jones Shults J, McDowell MR, et al. Anti-inflammatory effects of intravenously administered lidocaine hydrochloride on ischemia-injured jejunum in horses. Am J Vet Res 2009;70:1259–68.

46. Bauck AG, Grosche A, Morton AJ, et al. Effect of lidocaine on inflammation in equine jejunum subjected to manipulation only and remote to intestinal segments subjected to ischemia. Am J Vet Res 2017;78:977–89.

47. Montgomery JB, Hamblin B, Suri SS, et al. Remote lung injury after experimental intestinal ischemia-reperfusion in horses. Histol Histopathol 2014;29:361–75.

48. Daggett J, Grosche A, Abbott J, et al. Remote responses to intestinal ischemia and reperfusion injury in equine colon and jejunum. In: Proceedings of 12th International Equine Colic Research Symposium Lexington (KY): 2017, p. 39.

49. McCarthy GC, Megalla SA, Habib AS. Impact of intravenous lidocaine infusion on postoperative analgesia and recovery from surgery. A systematic review of randomized controlled trials. Drugs 2010;70:1149–63.

50. Ness TJ. Intravenous lidocaine inhibits visceral nociceptive reflexes and spinal neurons in the rat. Anesthesiology 2000;92:1685–91.

51. Robertson SA, Sanchez LC, Merritt AM, et al. Effect of systemic lidocaine on visceral and somatic nociception in conscious horses. Equine Vet J 2005;37: 122–7.

52. Cook VL, Jones Shults J, McDowell M, et al. Attenuation of ischaemic injury in the equine jejunum by administration of systemic lidocaine. Equine Vet J 2008;40: 353–7.

53. Fukuda H, Tsuchida D, Koda K, et al. Inhibition of sympathetic pathways restores postoperative ileus in the upper and lower gastrointestinal tract. J Gastroenterol Hepatol 2007;22:1293–9.

54. Nellgard P, Jonsson A, Bojo L, et al. Small-bowel obstruction and the effects of lidocaine, atropine and hexamethonium on inflammation and fluid losses. Acta Anaesthesiol Scand 1996;40:287–92.

55. Cassuto J, Jodal M, Tuttle R, et al. The effect of lidocaine on the secretion induced by cholera toxin in the cat small intestine. Experientia 1979;35:1467–8.

56. Larsson MH, Sapnara M, Thomas EA, et al. Pharmacological analysis of components of the change in transmural potential difference evoked by distension of rat proximal small intestine in vivo. Am J Physiol Gastrointest Liver Physiol 2008; 294(1):G165–73.

57. Bauck AG, Easley JT, Cleary OB, et al. Response to early repeat celiotomy in horses after a first surgery for jejunal strangulation. Vet Surg 2016;46:843–50.

58. Nolen-Walston R, Paxson J, Ramey DW. Evidence-based gastrointestinal medicine in horses: it's not about your gut instincts. Vet Clin North Am Equine Pract 2007;23:243–66.

59. Brianceau P, Chevalier H, Karas A, et al. Intravenous lidocaine and small-intestinal size, abdominal fluid, and outcome after colic surgery in horses. J Vet Intern Med 2002;16:736–41.

60. Torfs S, Delesalle C, Dewulf J, et al. Risk factors for equine postoperative ileus and effectiveness of prophylactic lidocaine. J Vet Intern Med 2009;23:606–11.

61. Salem SE, Proudman CJ, Archer DC. Has intravenous lidocaine improved the outcome in horses following surgical management of small intestinal lesions in a UK hospital population? BMC Vet Res 2016;12:157.

62. McKenzie JE, Beller EM, Forbes AB. Introduction to systematic reviews and meta-analysis. Respirology 2016;21:626–37.

63. Freeman DE, Hammock P, Baker GJ, et al. Short and long-term survival and prevalence of postoperative ileus after small intestinal surgery in the horse. Equine Vet J 2000;(Suppl 32):42–51.

64. Freeman DE, Schaeffer DJ. A comparison of handsewn versus stapled jejunocecostomy in horses - complications and long-term survival: 32 cases (1994-2005).

J Am Vet Med Assoc 2010;237:1060–7 [Erratum appears in J Am Vet Med Assoc 2011;238:65].

65. Freeman DE, Schaeffer DJ. Clinical comparison between a continuous Lembert pattern wrapped in a carboxymethylcellulose and hyaluronate membrane with an interrupted Lembert pattern for one-layer jejunojejunostomy in horses. Equine Vet J 2011;43:708–13.

66. Freeman DE, Schaeffer DJ, Cleary OB. Long-term survival in horses with strangulating obstruction of the small intestine managed without resection. Equine Vet J 2014;46:711–7.

67. Close K, Epstein KL, Sherlock CE. A retrospective study comparing the outcome of horses undergoing small intestinal resection and anastomosis with a single layer (Lembert) or double layer (simple continuous and Cushing) technique. Vet Surg 2014;43:471–8.

68. Smith MA, Edwards GB, Dallap BL, et al. Evaluation of the clinical efficacy of pro-kinetic drugs in the management of post-operative ileus: can retrospective data help us? Vet J 2005;170:230–6.

Fetal Membrane Removal in the Mare

Proactive Versus Reactive Approaches

Chelsie A. Burden, DVM, MS[a], Mark Meijer, DVM[b],
Malgorzata A. Pozor, DVM, PhD[c],
Margo L. Macpherson, DVM, MS[c],*

KEYWORDS

- Placenta • Retained fetal membranes • Mare

KEY POINTS

- The incidence of retained fetal membranes in mares is low, but the consequences can be severe.
- Prompt removal of retained fetal membranes is achieved through a variety of methods.
- Proactive removal of membranes (before retention) can be safely and effectively performed in normal, foaling mares and mares with retained fetal membranes.
- Fetal membrane weight contributes to increased incidence of postpartum complications such as uterine horn eversion and membrane retention.

INTRODUCTION

Retained fetal membranes (RFM) represent one of the more common postpartum problems in mares. Fetal membranes are considered retained in mares if they are not passed within 3 hours post partum.[1] Although the overall incidence is low (2%–10.6% of mares),[1,2] the consequences can be severe. Retained fetal membranes can lead to life-threatening sequelae such as metritis, sepsis, and laminitis.[1–4] Several factors are associated with a higher occurrence of RFM, including mare age, previous RFM, breed, and peripartum complications (abortion, dystocia, placentitis, prolonged gestation, and hydropic conditions).[1–5] However, the root cause for fetal membrane retention in mares is not clear. It has been hypothesized that a multitude of impaired physiologic changes lead to an abnormal release of the microvilli from the endometrial

Disclosure Statement: None.
[a] Goulburn Valley Equine Hospital, Congupna, Victoria 3633, Australia; [b] Dierenkiniek Zeddam, Zeddam NL7038 EP, the Netherlands; [c] Department LACS, College of Veterinary Medicine, University of Florida, Gainesville, FL 32610, USA
* Corresponding author. 2015 Southwest 16th Avenue, Gainesville, FL 32610.
E-mail address: macphersonm@ufl.edu

Vet Clin Equine 35 (2019) 289–298
https://doi.org/10.1016/j.cveq.2019.04.004
0749-0739/19/© 2019 Elsevier Inc. All rights reserved.

crypts in susceptible mares.[2] Allantochorion thickness, microvilli length, and degree of attachment at parturition along with an increased folding pattern of the nongravid horn are potential factors in increased membrane retention.[1] Fibrosis and adhesion formation have been reported in both microcotelydons and stromal connective tissue of heavy draft breeds, whereas low serum calcium concentrations have been directly linked to incidence of RFM in Friesian mares.[6–8] Recent information gathered in cows with RFM[9] showed reduced macrophage numbers (specifically CD172α) and altered caruncle proinflammatory cell trafficking in caruncular tissue. These findings suggest alterations in inflammatory responses that are critical to promoting release of placental tissue from the endometrium. It is not known if similar aberrations occur in mares with RFM.

Whatever the cause of retained membranes is for mares, the consequences can rapidly progress from mild (endometritis) to severe (metritis, laminitis, endotoxemia, death). Therefore, prompt expulsion of fetal membranes is a priority in the postpartum mare. There are clear advantages to actively removing membranes from mares at risk for retention or metritis (placentitis, dystocia, abortion). However, proactive membrane removal in the normal post-foaling period is a controversial topic in equine veterinary medicine.

Advantages of proactive membrane removal include the following:

- Reduced risk of metritis/endotoxemia/laminitis complex
- Reduced risk of uterine horn eversion (particularly in mares with heavy membrane)
- Full evaluation of the fetal membranes by the veterinarian
- Early institution of therapy in the case of membrane abnormalities

Potential risks of controlled membrane removal are as follows:

- Increased risk of hemorrhage when separating the microvilli from the endometrium
- Tearing membranes during removal, thus causing RFM
- Retained microvilli, which can provide a nidus for infection
- Uterine horn eversion/intussusception or prolapse.[1,3,10]

TRADITIONAL (REACTIVE) MEMBRANE REMOVAL TECHNIQUES

The most common reason for removal of equine fetal membranes is retention for a period of greater than or equal to 3 hours. A variety of methods to aid in removing retained membranes in the mare have been described.[1,5,11–13] The most common method to aid in fetal membrane removal is administration of oxytocin in the early postpartum period.[3,4] Oxytocin can be administered in bolus injections (5–20 IU, intravenously [IV] or intramuscularly [IM]) and repeated every 30 minutes to every 2 hours for the first 6 hours after foaling or until complete expulsion of the fetal membranes is achieved.[3,14] Alternatively, 60 to 100 IU oxytocin can be mixed in 1 L of lactated ringer solution or 0.9% saline solution and administered slowly (30–60 min), IV.[15] Uterine lavage is often combined with oxytocin administration to prompt membrane expulsion.[3] When the membranes are intact, the chorioallantois can be distended with dilute betadine solution or 0.9% saline[16] (Burns technique), which will stimulate release of microcotyledons from the endometrium. Fluid is infused into the chorioallantoic cavity, retained for a period of 15 to 30 minutes to facilitate membrane release and is siphoned out or expelled along with the intact membranes.

Alternatively, large volume uterine lavage is commonly used in both normal post-foaling mares and mares with retained membranes. Large volumes of fluid are infused directly into the uterus and around the membranes, with subsequent siphoning of the fluid from the uterus.[3,17] Six to twelve liters of warm saline (most often "homemade" by adding 3.5 ounces or 102 g of table salt to 12 L warm tap water) is infused into the uterus of postpartum mares using a sterile or clean nasogastric tube and stomach pump. This procedure allows for expansion of the uterus and rapid fluid removal. The fluid is actively siphoned, and the procedure is repeated for a total of 24 to 48 L or until the effluent character is relatively clear. At the time of fluid removal, care must be taken to prevent aspiration of retained membranes or endometrial tissue into the end of the tube. Large volume lavage facilitates expansion of the uterus, with possible detachment of microvilli, as well as removal of uterine debris and contaminants.

FACILITATED (PROACTIVE) MEMBRANE REMOVAL TECHNIQUES
Umbilical Vessel Infusion

Recently, a technique using catheterization of an exposed umbilical vessel to allow distension of membrane vasculature and detachment of the chorioallantois from the endometrium was described.[18] It was postulated that the chorionic microvilli stretch under fluid pressure causes separation of the fetal membranes from the endometrium. The weight of the fetal membranes concurrently increases during the procedure (with controlled support from the veterinarian), which also enhances the separation. Fluid often "leaks" into the space between the chorion and endometrium, thus facilitating further membrane separation. In the described study,[18] procedure was instituted in mares after administration of small, bolus injections of oxytocin failed to result in membrane expulsion. The procedure was described in both normal foaling mares and mares with RFMs.

To perform umbilical vessel catheterization, mares are restrained in stocks or in a stall. Immediately before the procedure, mares are administered oxytocin (10–20 IU, IM). A foal nasogastric tube or stallion catheter (with a maximum external diameter of 9 mm) is attached to a water hose using a hose connector with flow control valve (**Fig. 1**). An umbilical vessel (vein or artery, both are equally effective) is incised, longitudinally, using a standard scalpel blade (**Fig. 2**). The catheter, attached to the flow control fitting on the garden hose, is slowly advanced up the vessel under low water pressure until it cannot be advanced further (**Figs. 3** and **4**). The veterinarian manually holds the vessel closed around the tube (**Fig. 5**), or the vessel is secured to the tube using a zip tie. Slow to moderate water flow is used to infuse the vessel. The water flow

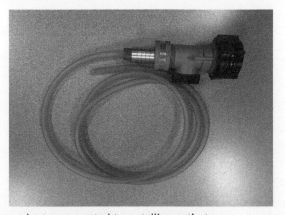

Fig. 1. Garden hose adapter connected to a stallion catheter.

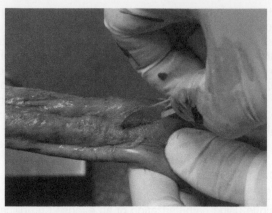

Fig. 2. Incising an umbilical vessel of the fetal membranes using a #10 scalpel blade.

is adjusted if the mare shows signs of discomfort or if there is significant fluid back flow. In mares showing mild discomfort (shifting weight, mild efforts to kick), fluid flow is discontinued for a short period to allow the mare to relax and to assess the progress of membrane release. If the membranes remain firmly attached, low-pressure fluid infusion is resumed. After 3 to 5 minutes of intravascular fluid infusion, gentle traction (using 2 fingers) is applied to the membranes at the mare's vulva to determine if the membranes easily separate from the endometrium and is external-ized. This procedure can be repeated in a circumferential fashion around the external membranes at the vulva to allow consistent separation of the membranes more prox-imally. Gentle traction is continued until the membranes are released (**Fig. 6**) or if the veterinarian determines that the membranes will not readily release. If the membranes remain tightly adhered, the procedure is discontinued to prevent injury to the mare or tearing of the membranes.

Using umbilical vessel infusion, the investigators reported[18] full separation and expulsion of fetal membranes in 92% (135/147) of mares within 5 to 10 minutes of initi-ating the procedure. Membrane expulsion occurred 15 to 30 minutes after infusion in 8 mares (5.4%). In 4 mares (2.7%), incomplete separation and tearing of the membranes

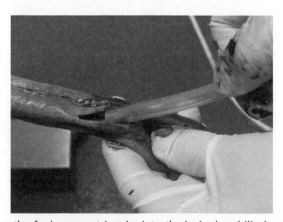

Fig. 3. Introducing the foal nasogastric tube into the incised umbilical vessel.

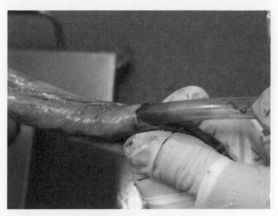

Fig. 4. The foal nasogastric tube is advanced up the umbilical vessel, using slight water pressure, until the tube can no longer be advanced.

occurred. All 4 mares had an unknown time from foaling to membrane removal, but it was estimated that membranes were retained for 12 to 24 hours after foaling. Eight mares (5.4%) showed mild signs of discomfort, comparable to the discomfort experienced by postpartum mares after oxytocin administration or mild colic. By reducing the water flow infusion rate, the mares became less painful. Other side effects to the procedure (inverted uterine horn, uterine prolapse, uterine artery hemorrhage, unresolvable colic, metritis) did not occur in any of the mares included in the data. In a subpopulation of 12 mares that were inseminated in the estrus after the procedure was performed, all 12 mares became pregnant on the first cycle of breeding.

The authors from this study, in addition to the clinical experience of the authors of this paper, find great utility for umbilical vessel infusion in the mare with membranes less than 8 hours old. Membranes after dystocia or prolonged retention begin to autolyze or suffer tissue damage, thus impairing vascular expansion. However, the procedure is easy and inexpensive to perform and carries little risk to the mare when performed properly. As a general rule, oxytocin administration is the first-line treatment to facilitate membrane removal. Umbilical vessel infusion is performed if the membranes do not release after oxytocin administration.

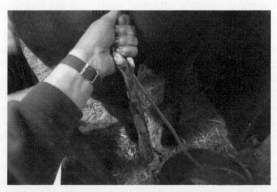

Fig. 5. The tube is held in place by the veterinarian while water is infused into the umbilical vessel for a period of 3 to 5 minutes.

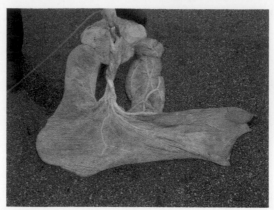

Fig. 6. The intact (edematous) placenta removed 10 minutes after water infusion of the umbilical vessel.

Controlled, Manual Removal of Fetal Membranes

Controlled, manual removal of fetal membranes is another proactive method of membrane removal that has been used for many years. Techniques that have been described for manual fetal membrane removal include grasping the externalized free portion of the membranes and applying controlled traction,[19,20] placing a hand between the endometrium and chorion to separate the attached membranes, twisting of the allantochorionic membrane into a tight cord,[21] and placing a wooden ring between the chorion and endometrium and advancing the ring to separate the membranes from the endometrium.[20]

A simple and safe method was described, in detail, with data supporting the use of the procedure.[22] This method of membrane removal is best performed with the mare standing or in sternal recumbency. Sternal recumbency is preferred because it eliminates the dependent weight of the membranes while performing the procedure. The mare's tail is wrapped and pulled laterally and the perineal area cleansed. Wearing a sterile examination glove, the veterinarian determines the degree of fetal membrane attachment to the endometrium through digital examination of the reproductive tract. Most often, the gravid horn is detached and free within the uterus, whereas the nongravid horn is attached to the endometrium. With a scissorlike action, 2 fingers are used to bluntly "dissect" the most caudally attached portion of the chorioallantois from the endometrium (uterine body and base of one or both horns; **Fig. 7**). With the base of the horns free from the endometrium, the membranes of the attached horn are encircled using the thumb and forefinger (**Fig. 8**). This "ring" of fingers is used in a gentle manner to move cranially up and back on the attached membranes to evenly separate the chorioallantois from the endometrium. The veterinarian is able to feel the chorionic attachment "peel" away from the endometrium while applying consistent, gentle pressure. Controlled pressure and digital separation of the placenta are repeatedly applied in a cranial direction toward the tip of the attached uterine horn. As membranes are separated from the endometrium, the "free" portion is exteriorized and transferred to the external hand (**Fig 9**). The external hand is used to relieve tension from the weight of the attached membranes to reduce the probability of membrane tearing or uterine horn eversion. This step is especially important for abnormally heavy membranes such as from mares with placentitis. Gentle detachment of the chorioallantois from the endometrium is continued as long as separation is easily performed. When the

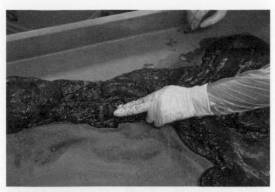

Fig. 7. Blunt dissection of the chorion using the 2-fingers scissorlike action. Endometrial surface not attached or pictured.

membranes stop detaching readily from the endometrium, the procedure should be discontinued and the mare reevaluated in 15 to 30 minutes. Manual detachment using a combination of 2-fingers scissorlike action to separate the membranes from the endometrium and gentle pressure up to the tip of the horn is continued for as long as progress is made detaching the membranes and the mare tolerates the procedure. The critical juncture occurs when the membranes are separated from the tip of the attached horn. Using careful dissection, the tip often can be "popped" off of the endometrium, intact. However, forceful pulling of the membrane tip, at this point, is discouraged, as this is the area where the membranes are most firmly attached. If forceful traction is applied to the remaining placental tip, the membranes can tear or the uterine horn can evert. Once the fetal membranes have been fully detached, they are exteriorized from the uterus and evaluated for completeness.

In a small study using a model of experimentally induced placentitis, the incidence of complications after using the described manual removal technique was compared with mares that spontaneously expelled their placentas. Two populations of mares were represented in the study: mares with experimentally induced bacterial placentitis and normal foaling mares. The incidence of uterine complications (horn eversion/prolapse) was not different (*P*>.05) after manual placental removal versus spontaneous placental expulsion in either mares with placentitis or normal foaling mares. Over all mares (placentitis and normal mares), fetal membranes were manually removed

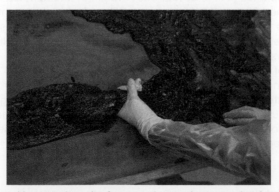

Fig. 8. "Ring" formed by encircling the free membranes between the thumb and forefinger. Endometrial surface not attached or pictured.

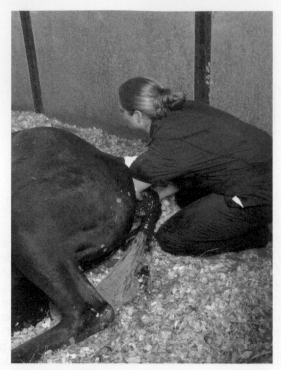

Fig. 9. Utilization of the free, external hand to alleviate the weight of the unattached, exteriorized membranes during manual removal.

from 12 of 17 mares, whereas 5 mares spontaneously delivered membranes. Membranes were manually removed without complications in 9 of 12 (75%) mares. Three mares whose membranes were manually removed (25%) suffered uterine horn eversion (n = 2) or uterine prolapse (n = 1). Five mares spontaneously expelled fetal membranes after delivery of the foal. Four of those five mares (80%) suffered complications (2 uterine horn inversion, 1uterine prolapse, 1 retained the tip of the nongravid horn). Most of the mares suffering complications after membrane delivery, independent of spontaneous expulsion or manual membrane removal, had placentitis and abnormally heavy fetal membranes (>11% of foal body weight).[23] Membranes from mares with placentitis weighed 20.1 ± 0.04% (mean ± SD) of foal body weight (kg) compared with membranes from normal foaling mares (10.6 ± 0.04%). This study concluded that placental weight played a significant role in postpartum complications such as uterine horn eversion/prolapse and retained membranes.

In all cases of manual placental removal techniques (umbilical vessel infusion; manual membrane removal), it is critical to evaluate the mare's reproductive tract to ensure that the uterine horns are not invaginated or that placental tags remain. Mares with RFM (≥3 hours after foal delivery) typically are treated with uterine lavage therapy and administration of therapeutic doses of oxytocin, antimicrobials, and flunixin meglumine or firocoxib, as needed.[3,24]

DISCUSSION

Manual removal of fetal membranes is a commonly used technique but has varying degrees of acceptance among equine veterinarians. Proponents of manual membrane removal cite advantages of rapid expulsion, thorough examination of membranes by a veterinarian, and reduced risk of retained membranes causing secondary complications. Potential risks of manual membrane removal are tearing and retention of fetal membranes, hemorrhage, and uterine horn eversion/uterine prolapse. The circumstances relevant to the mare (normal vs high risk pregnancy) and veterinarian (experience, access to the mare, breeding schedule) likely dictate the right decision for each mare. Essential to the decision-making process is a thorough knowledge of how to safely perform manual membrane removal to ensure the health of the mare. Risk factors that may negatively affect a mare if the membranes are not promptly removed contribute to the decision process.

Data from a model of experimental placentitis showed that abnormally heavy fetal membranes had a higher incidence of uterine horn eversion/prolapse or RFMs. This finding suggests a relationship between fetal membrane weight and uterine horn abnormalities postpartum, suggesting that controlled manual removal of fetal membranes may be advantageous.

The debate remains regarding the usefulness of controlled manual removal in normal foaling mares. The advantages of time saving and proper membrane evaluation for the attending veterinarian are clear. The methods described are quick and easily performed on a farm setting in experienced hands. Important to the discussion is recognizing an endpoint if the membranes are not released with controlled, gentle intervention. As a rule of thumb, membranes that are not released with 2 attempts (either umbilical infusion or manual removal) over the course of an hour should be left alone until a later time. At all times, the veterinarian should prioritize the well-being of the mare and institute only procedures that can be safely performed.

REFERENCES

1. Vandeplassche M, Spincemaille J, Bouters R. Aetiology, pathogenesis and treatment of retained placenta in the mare. Equine Vet J 1971;3:144–7.
2. Roberts SM. Veterinary obstetrics and genital diseases. Ithaca (NY): Woodstock; 1986.
3. Blanchard TL, Varner DD. Therapy for retained placenta in the mare. Vet Med 1993;88:55–9.
4. Frazer GS, Rossol TJ, Threlfall WR, et al. Histopathologic effects of dimethylsulfoxide on equine endometrium. Am J Vet Res 1988;49:1774–81.
5. Provencher R, Threlfall WR, Murdick PW, et al. Retained fetal membranes in the mare - a retrospective study. Can Vet J 1988;29:903–10.
6. Rapacz-Leonard A, Kankofer M, Leonard M, et al. Differences in extracellular matrix remodeling in the placenta of mares that retain fetal membranes and mares that deliver fetal membranes physiologically. Placenta 2015;36:1167–77.
7. Rapacz-Leonard A, Dabrowska M, Chmielewska-Krzesinska M, et al. Heavy mares that retain fetal membranes and those that deliver fetal membranes physiologically differ in production of PGF(2 alpha) and PGE(2). Reprod Domest Anim 2016;51:62.
8. Sevinga M, Barkema HW, Stryhn H, et al. Retained placenta in Friesian mares: incidence, and potential risk factors with special emphasis on gestational length. Theriogenology 2004;61:851–9.
9. Nelli RK, De Koster J, Roberts JN, et al. Impact of uterine macrophage phenotype on placental retention in dairy cows. Theriogenology 2019;127:145–52.
10. Hooper RN, Blanchard TL, Taylor TS, et al. Identifying and Treating Uterine Prolapse and Invagination of the Uterine Horn. Vet Med 1993;88:60–5.

11. Vandeplassche M, Spincemaille J, Herman J, et al. Twin pregnancy in the mare. Dtsch Tierarztl Wochenschr 1965;72:541–8 [in German].
12. Sevinga M, Barkema HW, Hesselink JW. Serum calcium and magnesium concentrations and the use of a calciumâ€"magnesium-borogluconate solution in the treatment of Friesian mares with retained placenta. Theriogenology 2002;57: 941–7.
13. Asbury AC. Management of the foaling mare. Proceedings for the international symposium on equine reproduction. 1974. p. 487–90.
14. Macpherson ML, Chaffin MK, Carroll GL, et al. Three methods of oxytocin-induced parturition and their effects of foals. J Am Vet Med Assoc 1997;210: 799–803.
15. Lamb CR, Koblik PD, O'Callaghan MW, et al. Comparison of bone scintigraphy and radiography as aids in the evaluation of equine lameness: Retrospective analysis of 275 cases, in Proceedings. Am Assoc Equine Pract 1989;35:359–68.
16. Burns SJ, Judge NG, Martin JE, et al. Management of retained placenta in mares. Proc Am Assoc Eq Prac 1977;23:381–90.
17. Brinsko S. How to perform uterine lavage: indications and practical techniques. Proceedings American Association of Equine Practitioners 2001;47:407–11.
18. Meijer M, Macpherson ML. How to use umbilical vessel water infusion to treat retained fetal membranes in mares. Proceedings American Association of Equine Practitioners 2015;61:478–84.
19. Cuervo-Arango J, Newcombe JR. The effect of manual removal of placenta immediately after foaling on subsequent fertility parameters in the mare. J Equine Vet Sci 2009;29:771–4.
20. Threlfall WR. Retained fetal membranes. 2nd edition. West Sussex (United Kingdom): Blackwell Publishing; 2001.
21. Rapacz A, Pazdzior K, Ras A, et al. Retained fetal membranes in heavy draft mares associated with histological abnormalities. J Equine Vet Sci 2012;32:38–44.
22. Burden C, Macpherson M, Pozor M, et al. How to utilize controlled manual removal of fetal membranes in mares. Proceedings American Association of Equine Practitioners 2018;64:240–4.
23. Whitwell KE, Jeffcott LB. Morphological studies on fetal membranes of normal singleton foal at term. Res Vet Sci 1975;19:44–55.
24. Canisso IF, Rodriguez JS, Sanz MG, et al. A clinical approach to the diagnosis and treatment of retained fetal membranes with an emphasis placed on the critically ill mare. J Equine Vet Sci 2013;33:570–9.

Update on Surgical Treatment of Wobblers

Lynn Pezzanite, DVM, MS[a], Jeremiah Easley, DVM[b],*

KEYWORDS

- Horse • Wobbler • Cervical vertebral compressive myelopathy

KEY POINTS

- Cervical vertebral compressive myelopathy (CVCM) is the most significant disease of the spinal cord in horses for which surgical treatment is described.
- Current surgical treatments for CVCM include ventral interbody fusion with kerf cut cylinders and dorsal laminectomy.
- Polyaxial pedicle screw and rod constructs and ventrally placed locking compression plate fixation represent alternative approaches to ventral interbody fusion.
- Advancements in advanced volumetric diagnostic imaging and endoscopy of the cervical vertebral canal may improve preoperative identification of locations of spinal cord compression to improve postoperative outcomes.
- Safety for return to athletic performance postoperatively should be evaluated on an individual basis with serial neurologic evaluations.

INTRODUCTION

Cervical vertebral compressive myelopathy (CVCM) represents the most significant disease of the spinal cord in horses for which surgical treatment is described. Intermittent or continuous extradural compression of the spinal cord results in substantial loss of athletic function.[1–4] CVCM presents clinically as a static or dynamic condition in either (1) young horses with multifactorial cause or (2) older horses where stenosis is attributed to osteoarthritis of the articular process joints. The most common presentation of CVCM is in young, rapidly growing horses. Narrowing of the cervical vertebral canal and malformation of cervical vertebrae or the surrounding ligamentous attachments result in compression of the spinal cord and subsequent neurologic deficits such as bilateral ataxia and weakness.

Disclosure Statement: The authors declare no conflicts of interest related to this report.
[a] Translational Medicine Institute, Department of Clinical Sciences, Colorado State University, 300 W Drake Road, Fort Collins, CO 80523, USA; [b] Preclinical Surgical Research Laboratory, Department of Clinical Sciences, Colorado State University, 300 W Drake Road, Fort Collins, CO 80523, USA
* Corresponding author.
E-mail address: easleyj@colostate.edu

Conservative medical management or surgical treatment of CVCM is described. As CVCM often results in significant loss of athletic function in equine patients intended for competition, the objective of surgical intervention is in many cases the return of athletic individuals to performance. Neurologic improvement postoperatively is determined individually by serial neurologic evaluation postoperatively, with some individuals never considered to be safe to handle or to carry a rider. For this reason, in addition to the reported high rate of complications in some studies, surgical intervention in the treatment of CVCM remains controversial. Despite these reservations, interest in optimization of surgical techniques to treat CVCM continues to increase, with the goal of improved safety and reduced postoperative complications.

DIAGNOSIS OF CERVICAL VERTEBRAL COMPRESSIVE MYELOPATHY

Diagnosis of CVCM may be made through collection and interpretation of the following clinical and diagnostic imaging findings:

- Patient history
- Physical examination
- Neurologic evaluation
- Diagnostic imaging
  - Radiographs of cervical spine
  - Myelography
  - Advanced volumetric diagnostic imaging of cervical spine (MRI, computed tomography [CT]) with or without contrast enhancement
- Cervical vertebral canal endoscopy

Neurologic examination reveals general proprioceptive deficits, with symmetric ataxia, paresis, dysmetria, and spasticity. Deficits are typically present in all 4 limbs but are frequently more noticeable in the pelvic limbs.

Standing lateral radiographs of the cervical vertebrae reveal bony malformations and suspected narrowing of the vertebral canal. However, the sensitivity and specificity of lateral cervical radiographs are limited by the assessment being restricted to the sagittal plane.[5] Furthermore, neck position influences some radiographic measurements of the cervical vertebrae in standing horses.[6] The intravertebral and intervertebral ratios calculated from cervical radiographs may be useful but require further validation. An intravertebral ratio of less than 0.5 was reported to increase the likelihood that cervical cord compression will be diagnosed by myelography at this site.[7] Another study evaluating these ratios against myelographic results demonstrated that the ratios were poor predictors of the site of compression but reasonably good predictors that the horse was likely to have a cervical compressive lesion somewhere within the cervical spine.[8] In the authors' experience in clinical practice, multiple sites are often fused to increase the odds of fusing the site where compression occurs, which is considered a controversial therapeutic plan. Improvement in diagnostic techniques to correct the site of compression may improve outcomes in the future.

Myelography, with either radiographic or CT evaluation, is considered essential to confirm diagnosis of CVCM, to determine sites of spinal cord compression, and to differentiate dynamic (type I) versus static (type II) lesions before surgical intervention. Narrowing or loss of the dorsal contrast column occurs at the site of compression (**Fig. 1**). Dynamic compressive lesions impinge on the spinal cord depending on cervical position, typically only visible in the flexed cervical spine, whereas static lesions

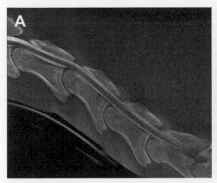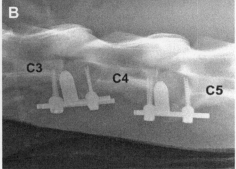

Fig. 1. (A) Myelogram with CT scan (sagittal view) of 3-year-old Quarter Horse gelding. Myelogram and CT revealed moderate compression at site C4-5 and mild compression at sites C3-4, C5-6, and C6-7 vertebrae in dynamic compression. (B) The patient underwent ventral interbody stabilization with polyaxial screw and rod constructs at sites C3-4 and C4-5.

impinge on the cervical spine regardless of position. Dynamic lesions are observed more frequently than static lesions.[9]

Advanced volumetric diagnostic imaging techniques (MRI, CT) of the cervical spine may represent one method to improve preoperative identification of sites of compression. Accurate diagnosis of cervical disease and identification of exact locations of spinal cord compression is imperative before surgical intervention but remains difficult in many cases. Recent studies emphasize the benefits of advanced imaging (CT, MRI) over plain radiographs.[5,10] MRI is considered the modality of choice for diagnosing cervical spinal pathology in other species[11,12]; however, the use of MRI is more limited in horses due to MR bore dimensions.

Few reports in the current literature describe CT and MRI of the equine cervical spine.[5,13–15] The normal anatomy of the equine cervical spine was recently described in detail comparing MR imaging and contrast-enhanced CT images in sagittal, dorsal, and transverse planes.[16] The anatomic location of clinically important structures including facet joints, spinal cord, cervical nerve roots and intervertebral discs were reliably identified in the anatomic sections and their corresponding MR images. Contrast-enhanced CT depicted all osseous borders, and MR images were superior for soft tissue imaging.[16] One recent comparison of MR imaging with standing cervical radiographs for evaluation of vertebral canal stenosis revealed that vertebral canal area and cord canal area ratio are better parameters to predict the location of cervical canal stenosis compared with only the sagittal plane of canal height.[5] Additional visual planes and measurements obtained by MRI, specifically vertebral canal area and cord canal area ratio, may provide a more accurate method to identify regions of canal stenosis than lateral cervical radiographs.[5] The development of MRI or CT equipment capable of evaluating the cervical column of mature live horses may substantially enhance evaluation of patients with CVCM (see **Fig. 1**). As appreciation of normal and abnormal equine cervical anatomy is improved, the usefulness of these imaging modalities in predicting clinical significance of cervical pathology will also likely increase.

Cervical vertebral canal endoscopy has been successfully used in humans as a technique to improve reliable identification of spinal cord compressions in CVCM, as well as to diagnose and treat several other conditions, including back pain.[17–21] Cervical vertebral canal endoscopy was recently reported in horses.[22] This technique involves introduction of a flexible videoendoscope via the atlantooccipital space into the epidural space or subarachnoid space and advancement to the level of the eighth cervical nerve. Anatomic structures identified included the dura mater, nerve roots, fat, and blood vessels in the epidural space and the spinal cord, blood vessels, arachnoid trabeculations, nerve roots, and the external branch of the accessory nerve in the subarachnoid space. Intraoperative complications reported with the procedure were mild and included increased mean arterial pressure during epiduroscopy. Postoperative complications included transient postoperative ataxia and muscle fasciculations following subarachnoid hemorrhage and air bolus in one horse undergoing myeloscopy. Analysis of the cerebrospinal fluid indicated mild inflammation on day 7 with values approaching normal by day 21. These results suggest that cervical vertebral canal endoscopy is relatively safe if performed correctly with rare postoperative side effects, and may allow more accurate identification of compression sites in horses with CVCM, and aid in diagnosis of other lesions within the cervical vertebral canal.[22] Prevalence of use of this technique in diagnosis of spinal cord compression at this time is unknown.

TREATMENT OF CERVICAL VERTEBRAL COMPRESSIVE MYELOPATHY

Current strategies for management of horses with CVCM include medical management or surgical procedures with the goal of stabilization of the vertebral joints at which compression is demonstrated with myelography (Table 1).

Medical management of horses with CVCM aims to reduce spinal cord swelling and edema formation with reduction of compression of the spinal cord. Treatments may include nonsteroidal antiinflammatory agents or corticosteroids in cases with acute spinal cord trauma. In young horses less than 1 year of age diagnosed with CVCM, a "controlled growth" program is recommended with restricted diet and activity.[23] Horses are maintained on stall rest with diets restricted in protein and carbohydrates while maintaining appropriate levels of vitamins and minerals in an attempt to slow growth to allow the vertebral canal diameter to "catch up" to the growth of the young horse.[24] In adult horses with compressive lesions of the spinal cord, options for medical therapy include stabilizing horses with acute neurologic deterioration by intraarticular injection of the cervical articular process joints with a combination of corticosteroids and polysaccharides (eg, hyaluronate sodium) to reduce soft tissue swelling and stabilize or prevent further bony proliferation. One retrospective study of Thoroughbreds showed that conservative management can result in approximately 30% return to racing.[25]

Surgical techniques for the treatment of equine CVCM were first introduced in 1979 and have been refined since that time. In general, 2 types of surgery that are advocated for the treatment of CVCM in horses are cervical stabilization with ventral interbody fusion or subtotal dorsal laminectomy.[1,26–32] Cervical stabilization through a ventral approach with ventral interbody fusion is most commonly used and represents a modification of the procedure developed by Cloward in 1958 for use in humans.[33] This method relies primarily on compression and does not provide stabilization in tension.[34–36] A stainless steel basket (Bagby basket) or kerf cut cylinder packed with autogenous bone graft is used for interbody fusion.[1,26,27,31,32,34] The procedure leaves a core of bone, the isthmus, to encourage growth of bone through the implant, and the remaining space is filled with autogenous bone graft. Complete bony fusion is expected to occur more rapidly by leaving the isthmus and its blood supply. Ventral interbody fusion with kerf cut cylinders may be used for any static and dynamic decompression, as it results in osseous remodeling of the articular processes and regression of associated soft tissue swelling at the treated site.

Table 1
Comparison of techniques in treatment of cervical vertebral compressive myelopathy

Technique	Advantages	Disadvantages
Medical Management For example, antiinflammatories, restricted diets, stall rest	• Effective in young horses less than 1 year of age • Least expensive treatment option	• Less effective in older horses or those with more severe lesions or multiple sites of compression
Surgical Techniques		
Dorsal laminectomy	• Appropriate technique in cases of intra- or extramedullary enlargement resulting in cord compression (eg, abscesses, granuloma, neoplasms)	• Difficult surgical approach • Long surgical time required; significant surgical expertise required to perform efficiently • Significant incidence of postoperative complications including articular facet fractures, compressive hematomas, and suppurative meningitis
Ventral interbody fusion Kerf cut cylinder (modification of originally described Bagby basket)	• Effectively provides compression between cervical vertebrae by encouraging boney fusion and stability • May be used for any static or dynamic compression	• Does not provide stabilization in tension
Locking compression plate	• Locking plate technology represents procedural advancement over previous ventral plating techniques • Effectively provides compression	• Complications reported include implant loosening, seroma, ventral screw migration, spinal cord injury, and plate breakage • Application limited by curved anatomic shape ventral vertebral body and restricted variability of locking screw placement
Pedicle screw and rod constructs	• Polyaxial screw head conforms to variable shape of ventral aspect of cervical vertebral bodies • No incidences of postoperative vertebral fracture or screw migration to date	• Implant loosening reported in one case • Limited use in veterinary market to date; more information on safety and outcomes will be available as become more accessible to veterinary market
Modifications of Surgical Techniques		
Modification of Seattle Slew surgical implants Enlargement of vertebral foramina Ventral compression kyphotic C2-3, C6-7, and C7-T1 with plating	• Clinical significance unknown at this time	

(continued on next page)

Table 1 (*continued*)		
Technique	**Advantages**	**Disadvantages**
Other Techniques		
Addition of regenerative therapies (mesenchymal stem cells) surrounding spinal cord	• Clinical significance unknown at this time	

Current techniques of surgical treatment of CVCM have been demonstrated to be beneficial in humans, dogs, and horses. In dogs with caudal cervical spondylomyelopathy, 89% showed improvement after surgical intervention.[24] In humans, 80% of patients with cervical spondylotic myelopathy and 80% to 90% patients with discogenic radiculopathy of the cervical spine showed improvement following anterior interbody fusion.[24] One report of 126 horses treated for CVCM with the KCC indicated that 77% of horses with CVCM showed improvement of neurologic deficits without complications, with 17% experiencing minor complications and 6% experiencing fatal complications.[37] Other studies in which the KCC was not exclusively used reported a wider range of success (43%–79%), with a fatal failure rate of up to 8%.[1,26,27,37–39] In general, young patients with mild clinical signs of short duration and single-site spinal cord compression have good prognosis for return to athletic function with surgery. It is estimated that more than 60% of such horses return to athletic function.[1,26,27] However, in the most recent case series of horses undergoing ventral cervical fusion, which was done primarily using the kerf cut cylinder technique, 57% of all horses that underwent ventral cervical fusion were eventually euthanized due to either vertebral body fracture or implant migration.[9] Based on these data, current surgical techniques for cervical fusion in horses still allow room for improvement in biomechanical stability and reduced rate of potentially fatal complications.

Alternative methods for ventral interbody fusion include the use of locking compression plates (LCP) and polyaxial pedicle screw and rod constructs.[40–42] Outcome of ventral fusion of 2 or 3 cervical vertebrae with LCPs was recently described in 8 horses.[38] Two or three cervical vertebrae were fused in 8 horses with median ataxia grade of 3/5 using either a narrow 4.5/5.0 LCP, broad 4.5/5.0 LCP, or a human femur 4.5/5.0 LCP plate. In this retrospective study, 2/8 horses required reoperation due to implant loosening, 6/8 developed seromas, 4/8 developed ventral screw migration, 1/8 developed spinal cord injury, and 2/8 horses experienced plate breakage.[38] Locking compression plates are effective for stabilization, but their application is limited by the pointed curved anatomic shape of the ventral vertebral body (known as the keel) and restricted variability of locking screw placement.[40,41] Stabilization via ventral compression of the cervical spine with LCPs is not optimal mechanically.[40,41] However, locking compression plate technology represents a procedural advancement over previous ventral plating techniques, with outcome considered excellent or good in 7/8 patients.[38]

The combination of an interbody fusion device (IFD) in conjunction with pedicle screws and connecting rods is currently considered the gold-standard technique for lumbar stabilization in humans[42] (**Fig. 2**). Pedicle screw and rod systems are used routinely in human spinal surgery and have experienced a resurgence of use in veterinary medicine.[43–47] Further attention has been focused on creating an improved IFD to be used in conjunction with pedicle screw stabilization.[42] The ideal IFD would allow for rapid growth of bone across the disc space to achieve full fusion quickly.[48–53] Various materials, ranging from acrylic and polyetheretherketone to metal alloys,

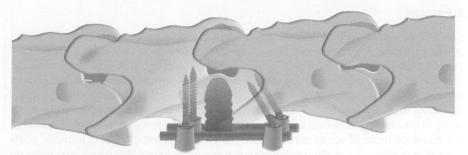

Fig. 2. Drawing of polyaxial pedicle screw and rod construct with screws placed on right and left side of ventral keel and placement of a porous metal interbody fusion device. (*Courtesy of* Kelsea Ericksen, Fort Collins, CO).

have been used to promote cervical stabilization in humans.[48–53] Polyaxial screw and rod constructs with a porous metal IFD were evaluated for feasibility and performance in 4 clinically normal horses in the stabilization of C3-C4 spinal units.[42] Evaluation of radiographs revealed no implant failure, implant migration, or spinal unit instability in any horses. The presence of new bone formation around the screw and rod constructs was confirmed via microCT. There was no histopathologic evidence of inflammation or iatrogenic damage. New bone was present within the interbody fusion device in all horses with variable osseointegration on the cranial and caudal surfaces of the implant at 8 months.[42]

The results of this preliminary work prompted evaluation of this technique in horses with diagnosis of cervical vertebral compressive myelopathy. To date, 10 clinical cases have been treated at Colorado State University with polyaxial screw and rod constructs, all with multisite stabilizations. Clinical trials are still ongoing, but estimated improvement in neurologic deficits and return to function for these horses is currently 65% to 70% (personal communication unpublished data, Dr Jeremiah Easley and Yvette Nout-Lomas, 2019). Preliminary results indicate that this technique may represent a safer alternative to current techniques of ventral interbody fusion with similar clinical outcomes. Further evaluation with increased patient numbers is indicated for more thorough comparison to current methods of ventral interbody fusion. The polyaxial screw head feature is an essential component for successful cervical stabilization in these clinical cases due to the variable shape of the ventral aspect of the cervical vertebral bodies. As these systems become more accessible to the veterinary market, they present a promising alternative to current surgical treatments for CVCM.

POSTOPERATIVE EVALUATION

Postoperatively, safety for performance should be evaluated individually on a case-by-case basis with serial neurologic evaluations. In horses, improvement of one neurologic grade minimum may be anticipated. However, appropriate education and discussion with owners and trainers of the risks, liabilities and assumed responsibilities associated with vertebral stabilization surgery is essential. Some individual horses may never be considered to be safe to handle or to carry a rider. For this reason, surgical intervention in the treatment of CVCM remains controversial. However, it is anticipated that further interest in optimization of surgical treatment for CVCM will continue with the goal of improved safety and reduced postoperative complications. Advances in preoperative diagnostic imaging and surgical techniques are anticipated to contribute to continued improvement in the treatment of equine CVCM.

SUMMARY

CVCM represents the most significant disease of the spinal cord in horses for which surgical treatment is described. Current surgical methods used include ventral interbody fusion with kerf cut cylinder and dorsal laminectomy. Polyaxial pedicle screw and rod constructs and ventral plating with locking compression plates have been introduced in the treatment of equine CVCM and present promising alternative approaches to ventral interbody fusion. Advancements in diagnostic imaging and endoscopy of the cervical vertebral canal may improve reliable preoperative identification of the exact locations of spinal cord compression in horses with CVCM to improve postoperative outcomes. Safety for performance postoperatively should be evaluated on an individual basis with serial neurologic evaluations.

REFERENCES

1. Moore B, Reed S, Robertson J. Surgical treatment of cervical stenotic myelopathy in horses: 73 cases (1983-1992). J Am Vet Med Assoc 1993;203:108–12.

2. Nixon A, Stashak T, Ingram J. Diagnosis of cervical vertebral malformation in the horse. Proc Am Assoc Equine Pract 1982;28:253–66.

3. Reed S, Newberry J, Norton K, et al. Pathogenesis of cervical vertebral malformation. Proc Am Assoc Equine Pract 1985;31:37–42.

4. Rooney JR. Disorders of the nervous system. In: Rooney JR, editor. Biomechanics of lameness in horses. 1st edition. Baltimore (MD): Wilkins & Wilkins; 1969. p. 219–33.

5. Janes JG, Garrett KS, McQuerry KJ, et al. Comparison of magnetic resonance imaing with standing cervical radiographs for evaluation of vertebral canal stenosis in equine cervical stenotic myelopathy. Equine Vet J 2014;46(6):681–6.

6. Beccati F, Santinelli I, Nannarone S, et al. Influence of neck position on commonly performed radiographic measurements of the cervical vertebral region in horses. Am J Vet Res 2018;79(10):1044–9.

7. Rush Moore B, Reed SM, Biller DS, et al. Assessment of vertebral canal diameter and bony malformations of the cervical part of the spine of horses with cervical stenotic myelopathy. Am J Vet Res 1994;55:5.

8. Luker M: The accuracy of minimum sagittal ratio values of standing lateral radiographs for the prediction of cervical vertebral myelopathy in horse. These for BSc (Hons) Diagnostic Radiography, 2005.

9. Szklarz M, Skalec A, Kirstein K, et al. Management of equine ataxia caused by cervical vertebral stenotic myelopathy: a European perspective 2010-2015. Equine Vet Educ 2018;30:370–6.

10. Kristoffersen M, Puchalski S, Skog S, et al. Cervical computed tomography (CT) and CT myelography in live horses: 16 cases. Equine Vet J 2014;46:11.

11. Alafifi T, Kern R, Fehlings M. Clinical and MRI predictors of outcome after surgical intervention for cervical spondylotic myelopathy. J Neuroimaging 2007;17: 315–22.

12. Da Costa RC, Parent JM. One-year clinical and magnetic resonance imaging follow-up of Doberman Pinschers with cervical spondylomyelopathy treated medically or surgically. J Am Vet Med Assoc 2007;231:243–50.

13. Moore BR, Holbrook TC, Stefanacci JD, et al. Contrast-enhanced computed tomography and myelography in six horses with cervical stenotic myelopathy. Equine Vet J 1992;24:197–202.

14. Claridge HAH, Piercy RJ, Parry A, et al. The 3D anatomy of the cervical articular process joints in the horse and their topographical relationship to the spinal cord. Equine Vet J 2010;42:726–31.

15. Mitchell CW, Nykamp SG, Foster R, et al. The use of magnetic resonance imaging in evaluating horses with spinal ataxia. Vet Radiol Ultrasound 2012;53:613–20.

16. Sleutjens J, Cooley AJ, Sampson SN, et al. The equine cervical spine: comparing MRI and contrast-enhanced CT images with anatomic slices in the sagittal, dorsal, and transverse planes. Vet Q 2014;34(2):74–84.

17. Uchiyama S, Hasegawa K, Homma T, et al. Ultrafine flexible spinal endoscope (myeloscope) and discovery of an unreported subarachnoid lesion. Spine 1998;23:2358–62.

18. Manchikanti L, Singh V. Epidural lysis of adhesions and myeloscopy. Curr Pain Headache Rep 2002;6:427–35.

19. Tobita T, Okamoto M, Tomita M, et al. Diagnosis of spinal disease with ultrafine flexible fiberscopes in patients with chronic pain. Spine 2003;28:2006–12.

20. Manchikanti L, Boswell MV, Rivera JJ, et al. [ISRCTN 16558617] A randomized, controlled trial of spinal endoscopic adhesiolysis in chronic refractory low back and lower extremity pain. BMC Anesthesiol 2005;5:10.

21. Warnke JP, Mourgela S. Adhesive lumbar arachnoiditis. Endoscopic subarachnoepidurostomy as a new treatment. Nervenarzt 2007;78:1182–7.

22. Prange T, Derksen FJ, Stick JA, et al. Cervical vertebral canal endoscopy in horse: intra- and postoperative observations. Equine Vet J 2011;43:404.

23. Mayhew IG, Donawick WJ, Green SL, et al. Diagnosis and prediction of cervical vertebral malformation in thoroughbred foals based on semi-quantitative radiographic indicators. Equine Vet J 1993;25(05):435–40.

24. Reed, Steven. Cervical vertebral stenotic myelopathy. Conference Proceedings, AO Advanced Techniques in Equine Fracture Repair, Columbus, OH, April 27–30, 2017.

25. Hoffman CJ, Clark CK. Prognosis for racing with conservative management of cervical vertebral malformation in Thoroughbreds: 103 cases (2002-2010). J Vet Intern Med 2013;27:317–23.

26. Grant BD, Barbee DD, Wagner PC, et al. Long-term results of surgery for equine cervical vertebral malformation. Proc Am Assoc Equine Pract 1985;31:91–6.

27. Walmsley J. Surgical treatment of cervical spinal cord compression in horses: a European experience. Equine Vet Educ 2005;17:39–43.

28. Nixon AJ, Stashak TS. Dorsal laminectomy in the horse I: review of the literature and description of a new procedure. Vet Surg 1983;12:172–6.

29. Nixon AJ, Stashak TS, Ingram JT. Dorsal laminectomy in the horse III: results in horses with cervical vertebral malformation. Vet Surg 1983;12:184–6.

30. Nixon AJ, Stashak TS, Ingram JT, et al. Dorsal laminectomy in the horse II: evaluation in the normal horse. Vet Sug 1983;12:177–83.

31. Wagner PC, Bagby GW, Grant BD, et al. Surgical stabilization of the equine cervical spine. Vet Surg 1979;8:7–12.

32. Wagner PC, Grant BD, Bagby GW, et al. Evaluation of cervical spinal fusion as a treatment in the equine "wobbler" syndrome. Vet Surg 1979;8:84–8.

33. Cloward RB. The anterior approach for removal of ruptured cervical disks. J Neurosurg 1958;15:602–17.

34. Grant GB, Bagby G, Rantanen N, et al. Clinical results of kerf cylinder (Seattle Slew Implant) to reduce implant migration and fracture in horses undergoing surgical interbody fusion. Vet Surg 2003;32:499.

35. Dukti SA, Robertson JT, Bertone AL, et al. Examination of an equine wobbler twelve years after surgical placement of a Bagby basket. Vet Comp Orthop Traumatol 2004;2:107–9.

36. Nout Y, Reed S. Cervical vertebral stenotic myeopathy. Equine Vet Educ 2003;15: 212–23.

37. Schutte A. Untersuchungen zym equinen wobbler syndrom. (Examination of the equine wobbler syndrome). Doctoral thesis. Munich (Germany): Ludwig-Maximilians-Universta; 2005.

38. Kuhnle C, Furst AE, Ranninger E, et al. Outcome of ventral fusion of two or three cervical vertebrae with a locking compression plate for the treatment of cervical stenotic myelopathy in eight horses. Vet Comp Orthop Traumatol 2018;31(5): 356–63.

39. Nixon AJ, Stashak TS. Surgical therapy for spinal cord disease in the horse. Proc Am Assoc Equine Pract 1985;31:61–74.

40. Reardon R, Kummer M, Lischer C. Ventral locking compression plate for treatment of cervical stenotic myelopathy in a 3-month-old warmblood foal. Vet Surg 2009;38:537–42.

41. Reardon RJ, Bailey R, Walmsley JP, et al. An in vitro biomechanical comparison of a locking compression plate fixation and kerf-cute cylinder fixation for ventral arthrodesis of the fourth and the fifth equine cervical vertebrae. Vet Surg 2010; 39:980–90.

42. Aldrich E, Nout-Lomas Y, Seim HB, et al. Cervical stabilization with polyaxial pedicle screw and rod construct in horses: a proof of concept study. Vet Surg 2018;47:932–41.

43. Smolders LA, Voorhout G, van de Ven R, et al. Pedicle screw-rod fixation of the canine lumbosacral junction. Vet Surg 2012;41:720–32.

44. Carpenter LG, Mann K, et al. Treatment of degenerative lumbosacral stenosis in military working dogs with dorsal laminectomy and pedicle screw and rod fixation. In: Proceedings of the American College of Veterinary Internal Medicine Forum. Charlottesville, NC, June 4–8, 2003. Abstract.

45. Meij BP, Bergknut N. Degenerative lumbosacral stenosis in dogs. Vet Clin North Am Small Anim Pract 2010;40:983–1009.

46. Meij BP, Suwankong N, Van der Veen AJ, et al. Biomechanical flexion-extension forces in normal canine lumbosacral cadaver specimens before and after dorsal laminectomy–discectomy and pedicle screw-rod. Vet Surg 2007;36:742–51.

47. Tellegen AR, Willems N, Tryfonidou MA, et al. Pedicle screw-rod fixation: a feasible treatment for dogs with severe degenerative lumbosacral stenosis. BMC Vet Res 2015;11:299.

48. Chou YC, Chen DC, Hsieh WA, et al. Efficacy of anterior cervical fusion: comparison of titanium cages, polyetheretherketone (PEEK) cages and autogenous bone grafts. J Clin Neurosci 2008;15:1240–5.

49. Epstein NE. Iliac crest autograft versus alternative constructs for anterior cervical spine surgery: pros, cons, and costs. Surg Neurol Int 2012;3:S143–56.

50. Jacobs W, Willems PC, van Limbeek J, et al. Single or double-level anterior interbody fusion techniques for cervical degenerative disc disease. Cochrane Database Syst Rev 2011;(1):CD004958.

51. Liao JC, Niu CC, Chen WJ, et al. Polyetheretherketone (PEEK) cage filled with cancellous allograft in anterior cervical discectomy and fusion. Int Orthop 2008; 32:643–8.

52. Niu CC, Liao JC, Chen WJ, et al. Outcomes of interbody fusion cages used in 1 and 2-levels anterior cervical discectomy and fusion: titanium cages versus polyetheretherketone (PEEK) cages. J Spinal Disord Tech 2010;23:310–6.

53. Shamji MF, Massicotte EM, Traynelis VC, et al. Comparison of anterior surgical options for the treatment of multilevel cervical spondylotic myelopathy: a systematic review. Spine 2013;38:S195–209.

Treatment Options for Melanoma of Gray Horses

Robert J. MacKay, BVSc (Dist), PhD

KEYWORDS

- Gray horse • Melanoma • Treatment • Vaccine • Immunotherapy

KEY POINTS

- All gray horses inherited a single gene mutation, $STX17^G$, that unbalances melanocyte behavior to cause graying and propensities to develop vitiligo and melanoma.
- The coat color genes $ASIP^a$ and $MC1R^E$ add risk such that relative likelihood of melanoma based on pregraying coat color is black > bay > chestnut.
- Melanomas begin at 4 years. Each year thereafter, prevalence increases 4% to 8%, and tumor severity in individual cases increases an average 0.1 to 0.3 grades (of 5).
- Locoregional control of melanoma masses depends on surgical removal and/or intralesional chemotherapy (possibly with adjunctive hyperthermia or electroporation).
- Systemic treatment is not evidence based but immunomodulators (cimetidine, levamisole) and vaccines can be tried.

INTRODUCTION

Ancient cultures venerated gray horses for their beauty and purity and their popularity continues to the present day.[1] A single gene mutation (aka the "gray gene") that occurred more than a millennium ago is inherited by all gray horses and controls not only the coat color but also the propensity for the development of melanomas.[1,2] Presumably, the association between gray coat and melanoma has long been recognized but it was not described until 1903.[1] Paradoxically, despite the considerable progress made in understanding the molecular events underlying graying, relatively little headway has been made in understanding and managing the associated clinical challenges of gray horse melanoma.

WHAT IS THE GRAY GENE?

The mutation causing graying has been localized to a single 4.6-kb duplication in intron 6 of the syntaxin-17 (STX17) gene.[1] This region contains a cis-acting

Disclosure Statement: Nothing to disclose.
Department of Large Animal Clinical Sciences, University of Florida, PO Box 100136, Gainesville, FL 32610, USA
E-mail address: mackayr@ufl.edu

Vet Clin Equine 35 (2019) 311–325
https://doi.org/10.1016/j.cveq.2019.04.003
0749-0739/19/© 2019 Elsevier Inc. All rights reserved.
vetequine.theclinics.com

melanocyte-specific enhancer that is upregulated by duplication.[3] The gray-inducing *STX17* duplication boosts expression of *STX17* and its neighboring gene *NR4A3* to higher than normal levels. Although it is still unclear precisely how these upregulated genes cause graying and associated phenotypic effects, it has been proposed that the key outcome is enhanced melanocyte proliferation.[1] In hair follicles, melanocytes are recruited from a finite pool of stem cells that normally are progressively depleted during each round of hair growth and shedding.[1,4,5] Overproliferation of melanocytes in gray horses likely prematurely exhausts the stem cell supply, leading to progressive pileous depigmentation and graying.[1] In contrast, enhanced proliferation of dermal and epidermal melanocytes in hairless skin may predispose melanocytes to neoplastic transformation and formation of melanomas. Consistent with the notion that *STX17* mutation (*STX17^G*) is a melanoma-driving element, *STX17^G* copy number expansions were found in 5 of 8 melanoma sources, with a tendency toward highest copy number in aggressive tumors.[2]

WHAT ARE THE PHENOTYPIC EFFECTS OF THE GRAY GENE?

The gray-inducing duplication mutation *STX17^G* (G) is both autosomal dominant and epistatic for coat color, that is, horses of any base color (black, bay, chestnut) with *STX17^G* at one or both alleles (ie, G/g or G/G) will become gray.[3] *STX17^G* strongly influences *four* different age-related phenotypic traits: gray coat color, melanoma, vitiligo, and speckling of the gray coat. In 2 large studies of gray Lipizzaners, the narrow-sense heritabilities (ie, the proportion of total phenotypic variance explained by total *additive* genetic variance) of melanoma occurrence were 0.36 and 0.37.[3,6] Despite the moderate heritability of each of these traits, there is substantial variation among individuals as to the rate and completeness of the graying process and the prevalence and progression of the other traits. Some of this variation is explained by the modulating effect of *STX17^G* copy number. Compared with heterozygotes, horses with the G/G genotype gray more quickly and completely and have greater prevalence and severity of melanomas, more vitiligo of hairless skin, and less speckling of the gray coat. For example, for a cohort of 1119 Gy Lipizzaner horses, the estimated effect of an additional *STX17^G* copy on melanoma grade (out of 5) for homozygotes compared with heterozygotes was 0.85 grades.[3]

DO OTHER COAT COLOR GENES AFFECT MELANOMA OCCURRENCE IN GRAY HORSES?

The base coat colors of horses—namely, black, bay, and chestnut—are controlled predominantly by 2 gene loci, *Extension* and *Agouti*. The wild-type alleles at *Extension* and *Agouti* are *MC1R^E* (encodes melanocortin-1 receptor) and *ASIP^A* (encodes agouti signaling protein), respectively. The dominant *MC1R^E* allele enables synthesis of the black hair pigment eumelanin, and in the presence of at least one copy of *MC1R^E*, the *ASIP^A* allele is dominant for restriction of black hair to the body extremities with resultant bay coat pattern. Recessive alleles at the *Extension* and *Agouti* loci are loss-of-function mutations *MC1R^e* and *ASIP^a*, respectively. Horses that are e/e do not synthesize eumelanin but instead only produce the red pigment pheomelanin and have chestnut coat color. In the context of at least one copy of *MC1R^E*, horses that are a/a have a uniformly black coat. Thus, black horses have the genotype E/-, a/a; bay horses are E/-, A/-; and chestnuts are e/e, −/−, where (−) stands for either the dominant or the recessive allele. Agouti signaling protein reduces MC1R activation by interfering with the binding of alpha-melanocyte-stimulating hormone (α-MSH), whereas horses with mutant *ASIP* do not have this inhibition. Because the *STX17^G* mutation and signaling through MC1R both promote melanocyte proliferation, unrestricted activation of MCR1 in horses with the $ASIP^a$ mutation may be expected to enhance melanoma development. In a large study of melanoma in gray Lipizzaners, the estimated effect on melanoma grade was 0.19 grades (out of 5) per copy of the mutated *ASIP* gene; thus, melanoma grade in *a/a* homozygotes was an estimated 0.38 grades higher than in *A/A* horses.[3] By the same logic, it is obvious that the $MC1R^e$ mutation should lower melanoma risk.[4] Because of the very low prevalence of chestnut coat color in Lipizzaners, this hypothesis could not be tested.[3] Based on the foregoing, the relative risk for melanoma based on pregraying coat color is hypothesized to be black > bay > chestnut (**Fig. 1**).

WHAT IS MELANOMA OF GRAY HORSES?

A melanoma results from an abnormal proliferation of melanocytes, usually appearing as one or more nodules. Melanocytes are specialized cells of neuroectodermal origin with precursors that migrate widely through the body and colonize the epidermis and hair bulbs.[5] In a process involving engagement of melanocortin-1 receptors by α-MSH, intracellular production of cAMP, and the actions of tyrosinase, melanin pigments, both black-brown *eumelanin* and red-yellow *phaeomelanin*, are synthesized from tyrosine substrate and packaged in melanosomes. Melanosomes are transferred to keratinocytes and hair shafts to provide skin and hair color. Most of the dermal melanomas in gray horses appear as pigmented (black to gray) hemispheric to ovoid dermal nodules or plaques that may be solitary, in clusters, or multicentric involving widely separated cutaneous sites.

HOW COMMON ARE MELANOMAS?

Melanomas in gray horses are very common. In surveys of gray horses that include all age groups, the prevalence of melanomas has ranged from 16% of the Quarter Horse breed to 31% of Camargue horses and 50% of Lippizanners.[4] Melanomas typically first appear in a group of gray horses at 4 to 8 years of age, and the proportion of affected horses then increases approximately linearly by 4% to 8% annually until at

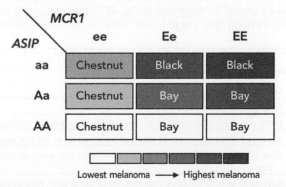

Fig. 1. Association among mutations of *ASIP* and *MC1R*, coat color, and risk of melanoma. The melanoma risks shown are based on the reported additive effect of *ASIP* mutation on melanoma grade[3] and a hypothesized additive effect of *MCR1* mutation on melanoma grade. (*From* Teixeira RBC, Rendahl AK, Anderson SM, et al. Coat color genotypes and risk and severity of melanoma in gray quarter horses. Journal of Veterinary Internal Medicine 2013;27:1201–1208; with permission)

least 20 years of age.[4,7,8] In gray horses older than 15 years, the prevalence of melanomas was 51% in Quarter horses, 68% in Camargue horses, and 78% in Lipizzaners.[3,4,7]

ARE MELANOMAS MALIGNANT?

Although melanomas in horses of all colors are variable in appearance and behavior on a continuum from sessile nevi to aggressively invasive metastatic multicentric tumors, those in gray horses usually begin as one or several nodules that are black on cross-section. From the earliest stages, these tumors display subtle nuclear and cellular atypia (eg, presence of nucleoli and variations in shape, size, and nuclear/cytoplasmic ratio), which suggests cancerous potential, although mitotic figures are rare.[9] Rather than being classified as benign, early melanomas should therefore be considered precancerous, with the potential to grow and progress to malignancy.

DO MELANOMAS SHORTEN THE AVERAGE LIFESPAN OF GRAY HORSES?

Although some gray horses certainly die because of melanoma, there are no reliable data that quantify the "gray effect" on longevity. Virtually all Lipizzaner horses are gray and about 80% of those older than 15 years have melanoma, yet this breed is notably long-lived with reported average lifespan of 30 to 35 years. A study[10] often cited as evidence for shortened lifespan of gray horses compares nonmatched cohorts of gray and nongray Thoroughbred mares from the mid-nineteenth century and only finds high death rate in gray horses younger than 10 years, a finding unlikely to be explained by the effects of melanoma.

WHAT IS THE PROGNOSIS FOR GRAY HORSES WITH MELANOMA?

Over a period of many years, melanomas in gray horses are thought to advance through the stages shown in **Table 1** to possibly progress into serious locoregional malignancy in stage 4, then clinical complications and physical decline in stage 5. In surveys of gray horses with melanomas there is an approximately linear relationship between age and tumor stage. For example, across a group of 47 Old Kladruber horses with melanomas, mean melanoma stage was about 0.15 higher for each year between ages 7 and 21 years[9] (orange line in **Fig. 2**). Thus, assuming that there is also linear progression through the stages over time in individual horses, these data

Table 1	
Clinical classification of melanoma grade	
Grade	**Description**
0	Free of melanoma
1	Early stage of plaque type of single 0.5-cm nodule at typical locations
2	Several 0.5-cm nodules, or single 2-cm nodule, at typical locations
3	One or several nodules of 5 cm intra- or subcutaneous at typical locations or lips
4	Extensive confluent subcutaneous melanoma with necrosis or ulceration, metastasis
5	Exophytic tumor growth, with wet surfaces and ulceration, metastasis to organs with associated clinical signs (cachexia, fever, metabolic disorders)

Adapted from Curik I, Druml T, Seltenhammer M, et al. Complex inheritance of melanoma and pigmentation of coat and skin in Gray horses. *PLoS Genet* 2013; with permission.

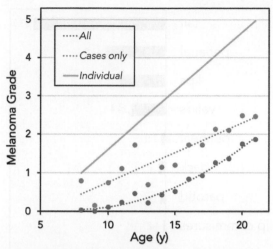

Fig. 2. Effects of age on melanoma grade in a population of gray Old Kladruber horses. Blue circles are mean grade for all horses in the population (ie, those with and those without melanomas). Orange circles are calculated mean grade for cases (ie, horses with melanomas), and the green line is the hypothesized average progression through the melanoma grades of a horse first diagnosed with grade 1 melanoma at age 8 years. The data for all horses are from Hofmanova and colleagues,[8] 2015, and the data for cases (and individual progression rate) are calculated from the prevalence information in Hofmanova and colleagues, 2015. (*Data from* Hofmanova B, Vostry L, Majzik I, et al. Characterization of greying, melanoma, and vitiligo quantitative inheritance in Old Kladruber horses. Czech Journal of Animal Science 2015;60:443–451.)

suggest that melanomas in individual Old Kladruber horses can be expected to advance an average 0.3 stages per year (see **Fig. 2**). It is therefore reasonable to expect an 8-year-old horse with newly developed stage 1 melanoma to cross the threshold to stage 4 in 10 years (ie, at age 18 years) and to suffer the life-threatening effects of stage 5 two to three years later. Similar rates of melanoma progression are reported for horses of other breeds selected for gray coat color, such as the Lipizzaner and Camargue horse.[1,3,7] The melanomas of 56 gray horses of a breed, the Quarter horse, not usually selected for this coat color, showed comparatively slow average growth of 0.057 stages per year, with an expected average progression in individual horses of only 0.11 stages annually, or 8 to 9 years per stage.[4] Note that the abovementioned are modeled rates of progression based on average data for large numbers of horses; actual rates of progression differ among individual horses and over time.

WHAT ARE THE CLINICAL SIGNS OF MELANOMA IN GRAY HORSES?

The clinical presentation of melanoma in gray horses has been reviewed[6,7,11–13] and are summarized here. Most melanomas present initially as single, small, raised black cutaneous nodules or plaques in an area of glabrous (hairless) skin. In one survey of tumor locations in gray Camargue horses with melanomas, more than 90% of affected horses had at least one tumor on the ventral aspect of the tail (**Fig. 3**). Perianal and perineal melanomas were also common.[7] Nodules likewise occur commonly on the prepuce and penis, commissures of the lips, around the eyes, and within or around the parotid salivary glands.[6,9] The rates of progression of melanomas are highly

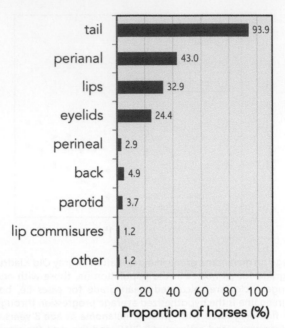

Fig. 3. Locations of tumors in a population of gray horses with melanomas. (*Adapted from* Fleury C, Berard F, Leblond A, et al. The study of cutaneous melanomas in Camargue-type gray-skinned horses (2): Epidemiologic survey. Pigment Cell Research 2000;13:47–51; with permission.)

variable and progression likely occurs in stop-start fashion. With advancement through the melanoma stages, the tumor burden increases in some to all of the following ways, in approximate ranking of frequency: enlargement of the original masses, development of adjacent, sometimes coalescing nodules (satellitosis), appearance of new cutaneous or deep masses along the lymphatic drainage systems of existing tumors (in-transit metastasis), new cutaneous masses at distant sites, and deep tissue/visceral tumors. Progression likely involves some combination of (1) spread of existing tumors via local, lymphatic, or vascular spread and (2) emergence of new generations of primary melanomas at cutaneous or internal sites. Unfortunately, the relative contribution of these 2 processes is completely unknown.

As dermal and subcutaneous tumor masses enlarge and coalesce, there may be anatomic disruption of vital functions and performance. For example, perianal and perirectal masses cause dyschezia and rectal impaction; preputial and penile masses interfere with penile intromission during breeding; vulval melanomas affect breeding and parturition; melanomas involving the parotid salivary glands and proximal neck cause discomfort under the crownpiece and throatlatch of the bridle and interfere with flexion and other head movements; and masses around the pharynx or larynx interfere with eating, drinking, or breathing. Masses that are continually rubbed by either tack or the tail may ulcerate leading to exacerbation of clinical signs. Visceral and deep tissue masses may affect organ function and cause systemic signs. Epidural and perineural melanomas have caused a variety of neurologic signs, and accumulation of splenic, pulmonary, lymph node and/or hepatic tumors ultimately results in inappetence, colic, fever, and/or weight loss. The cores of rapidly growing individual tumor masses outgrow vascular supplies and can become acutely necrotic and present signs of sterile abscessation (local heat and pain, fever), before rupturing and discharging black tarry contents onto the skin.

HOW IS MELANOMA OF GRAY HORSES TREATED?

The quality of data regarding gray horse melanoma is uniformly low because of small numbers of horses treated and heterogeneity of treatment protocols. Most insights are drawn from studies of human or canine malignant melanoma, which biologically are very different from equine melanoma. The following is not a comprehensive listing of equine melanoma treatments but focuses on approaches supported by multiple equine studies and/or sound conceptual bases.

Surgical Excision

Surgical removal of tumor masses is the mainstay of melanoma treatment of gray horses. In some cases, cryotherapy or CO_2 laser surgery is used to replace or supplement traditional surgical methods. Where necessary, cisplatin or carboplatin beads or slow-release emulsions are used to infiltrate tissue margins not fully accessible to surgical excision. When surgical margins are clear microscopically, or even grossly, tumor regrowth at the site of excision is unlikely, even over a period of years. In a recently reported case series, 38 melanomas ranging from 4 to 20 cm diameter were removed surgically.[14] Some of the tumors were necrotic and ulcerating (ie, stage 3 or 4[8]) and several involved a parotid salivary gland; some could not be closed primarily and were allowed to heal by second intention. None regrew at the excision site during the 12 to 163 months of follow-up. There is a common perception that melanomas have a tendency to regrow aggressively at the site of surgical removal, yet virtually no specific evidence is offered for this claim.[11,13] Not surprisingly, surgical removal of a melanoma does not seem to affect the continued growth of the remaining tumor masses.[14]

Intratumoral Cytotoxic Drugs

As sole modality: although melanoma cells are relatively resistant to the concentrations of cytotoxic chemotherapeutic agents that can be achieved systemically, intratumoral treatment with the platinum-based agents, cisplatin and carboplatin, can be effective.[15] The cytotoxic drugs bleomycin and 5-fluorouracil have proved useful against squamous cell carcinoma and sarcoid in horses but have not found a place in melanoma treatment. Carboplatin is an analogue of cisplatin; both drugs act by cross-linking DNA of tumor cells. Although cisplatin and carboplatin are considered bioequivalent, comparative studies of efficacy in melanomas of gray horses have not been performed. Either drug is prepared for intratumoral injection as a 3.3 mg/mL emulsion by "push-pull" mixing of 10 mg/mL aqueous solution with sesame seed oil (1:2 ratio).[15,16] Sorbitan monooleate and epinephrine can be added to the mixture to improve emulsion characteristics and increase drug dwelling times.[16] The emulsion is injected via 22-gauge needles inserted along parallel tracks and, if necessary, across multiple tissue planes, such that adjacent tracks are spaced at 1-cm intervals through and around the tumor. This procedure is designed to deposit 0.3 mL emulsion containing 1 mg drug per cubic centimeter of tumor. Although the oil component is intended to promote retention of the drug, it also causes inflammation, and some investigators prefer to use unaltered aqueous solutions of carboplatin (usually at 1 mg/mL).[12] One to four treatments are given at 2-week intervals. Of 16 melanomas less than or equal to 5 cm diameter that were treated with intratumoral cisplatin in this manner, 14 (87.5%) were eliminated and recurrence free for at least

2 years. Cisplatin and carboplatin may also be formulated into biodegradable beads (eg, 1.6 mg cisplatin or 4.6 mg carboplatin per 3-mm diameter bead) and surgically inserted subcutaneously alongside small (≤1.5 cm) cutaneous melanoma nodules.[17] Two nodules treated this way resolved without recurrence for at least 2 years.[17] Because platinum-based agents are mutagenic and carcinogenic, strict safety rules must be observed during all phases of preparation and use.[18]

As adjuvant to surgery

Tumors larger than about 2 cm diameter are usually removed or debulked surgically. If surgical margins are not clear, then cisplatin or carboplatin emulsion or biodegradable beads can be introduced into the wound margins either intraoperatively or after histologic results become available. Emulsions are injected as described in the previous section at intervals of 1 cm, whereas beads are sutured into pockets created every 1.5 to 2 cm around the wound margins and into the wound bed of open wounds.[14,15,17] None of the 10 large melanomas (ie, grade 3 or greater) treated with surgical debulking and cisplatin beads recurred during the 12 months after surgery.[14]

With adjunctive procedures to enhance cytotoxicity

Electrochemotherapy. Electrochemotherapy (ECT) is a relatively new procedure that combines transient tumor permeabilization with the use of chemotherapeutic agents.[19] Electrical pulses are applied across tumors to open transient pores in cell membranes and propel drug molecules into the cytosol. Because of heightened intracellular dose intensity, the cytotoxicity of bleomycin is increased up to 8000-fold and that of cisplatin is boosted up to 80-fold. ECT also drives cytotoxic agents into endothelial and stromal cells, thereby disrupting the blood supply and structure of the treated tumor. The procedure in horses is performed under sedation or general anesthesia immediately after saturation of the tumor with aqueous cisplatin or carboplatin (1 mg/mL), as described earlier. ECT has been applied successfully to the treatment of sarcoids of horses[20,21] and is beginning to be used to treat melanomas.[22,23] Because standard electropulsators are only effective to a depth of 1 cm, ECT should be reserved for small tumors or combined with surgical debulking of larger tumors.[21]

Hyperthermia. Targeted hyperthermia of tumors potentially produces or enhances antitumor effects along multiple pathways.[24] When the tumor and surrounding tissues are heated to 41 C to 43 C, tumor cells (but not normal cells) are subjected to heat stress, causing overexpression of heat shock proteins and shedding of molecules that express damage-associated molecular patterns, thereby boosting innate and acquired antitumor immune responses. Heat also enhances the cytotoxicity of chemotherapeutic agents by reversibly permeabilizing cell membranes and suppressing DNA repair mechanisms. Tumor tissue can be effectively heated using ultrasound, radiofrequency, or microwave energy.[12] One relatively simple commercially available system (ThermoField 250A system; Thermofield, Franklin, TN) uses microwave energy to heat tissues under a large application plate to a depth of several centimeters.[12] It is recommended that 2 rounds of 30 to 60 minutes of hyperthermia are delivered after intratumoral cisplatin or carboplatin, with treatment repeated every 2 weeks as necessary. This technique is applicable to debulked tumors but also was effective in completely resolving melanomas without surgery on 2 horses, one of which was "an extremely large tail-base tumor."

Radiation

The use of ionizing radiation to treat cancer is well established in human and small animal medicine. Radiotherapy has so far found limited application to horse cancers, however, and typically is restricted to irradiation of small tumors in and around the eyes.[25] Because melanomas of humans and dogs are considered relatively radioresistant and delivery of radiation therapy to horses is specialized and expensive, this modality is seldom used for treatment of gray horse melanomas. Nonetheless, there are situations where radiotherapy can be applied to horses with melanomas.

Palliation of the effects of large inaccessible melanomas
This typically involves teletherapy to shrink multiple large masses around the head and proximal neck, some of which may only be discovered by computed tomography.[26] Teletherapy refers to the use of radiation from an external source, usually cobalt 60 or a linear accelerator.[25] The total prescribed dose (eg, 30–45 Gy) is given in fractions over several sessions, each under general anesthesia.

Treatment of cutaneous tumors unresponsive or inaccessible to other modalities
Radiotherapy for this purpose usually is provided by brachytherapy. Brachytherapy involves placement of a radiation source within, or in contact with, the tumor target. Traditionally, radioactive isotopes, such as iridium-192 or strontium-90, have been used, with the attendant requirements for shielded housing and other safety precautions. A practical alternative to this approach is the use of electronic brachytherapy, which delivers radiation to the tumor via a miniaturized electrically powered x-ray source. A device of this type (Xoft AXXENT Ebx System; Xoft, San Jose, CA, USA) was used to successfully treat an extensive preputial melanoma in a gray horse.[27]

Immunotherapy

It is increasingly recognized that the immune system is critical in preventing the development and progression of cancer and that subversion of this immune surveillance is a defining characteristic of "successful" cancers.[28] Much of the substantial recent improvement in overall survival of humans with metastatic melanoma can be attributed to innovative treatments that seek to directly boost anticancer immune function and/or prevent tumor-mediated suppression of immunity. The application of modern immunotherapy strategies to canine melanomas has recently been reviewed.[28] Approaches include nonspecific activation of innate and adaptive immunity, inhibition of inactivation pathways, monoclonal antibodies against tumor antigens, vaccines, and oncolytic viruses. The following are summaries of equine immunotherapy approaches to melanoma.

Nonspecific stimulation of immunity
Bacillus Calmette-Guerin (BCG), a live attenuated strain of *Mycobacterium tuberculosis*, is the prototypic immunostimulant.[15] This group of agents, which includes killed *Propionibacterium acnes* and purified mycobacterial cell wall components, contain pathogen-specific molecular patterns that act through specific cellular receptors (eg, toll-like receptors) to cause release of inflammatory cytokines and other molecules. Intravesical BCG is the treatment of choice for bladder cancer in humans, but BCG, given subcutaneously, intradermally, or intralesionally, has failed to show benefit in metastatic melanoma of humans.[29] Although intralesional BCG is quite effective in treatment of equine sarcoids, there are no reports of similar success with treatment of melanomas in horses.

Interleukin (IL) 12 and IL-18 are cytokines that stimulate multiple processes at the nexus of the innate and acquired immune responses. Equine melanomas were injected 1 to 6 times, with DNA vectors loaded with genes encoding either human IL-12,[30] equine IL-12,[31] equine IL-18,[31] or a combination of equine IL-12 and IL-18.[32] In each instance, there was significant reduction in volume of injected tumors—approximately 20% for equine genes[31,32] and 60% for human IL-12.[30] In horses given the IL-12/IL-18 combination, the DNA vector was also administered intramuscularly and in those horses tumor shrinkage was also found in noninjected melanomas.[32]

Control of tumor immunosuppression

The tumor microenvironment is profoundly immunosuppressive. Regulatory T lymphocytes (Tregs), tumor-associated M2 macrophages, and myeloid-derived suppressor cells contribute to tumor progression by suppressing normal immune responses and thwarting the actions of antitumor vaccines and other immunotherapies.[24] Recently, monoclonal antibodies have been developed that target the immunosuppression characteristic of human melanomas. These monoclonal antibodies (mAbs) enhance the activity of intratumoral cytotoxic T cells by blocking key checkpoint inhibitor molecules.[28,33] One traditional approach to melanoma treatment of horses, cimetidine, has found continued application in tumor therapy regimens in human medicine, likely because of its ability to inhibit the suppressive action of Tregs.[34,35] Cimetidine, used as monotherapy, at doses of 1.6 to 7.5 mg/kg/daily has been reported to achieve long-term melanoma involution in some horses in a few early reports,[36–38] but no obvious effect was found in most of the follow-up case series.[39] These reports of occasional responses to cimetidine should not be dismissed for the following reasons: (1) spontaneous regression of melanomas of gray horses is a vanishingly rare phenomenon, so any credible report of tumor shrinkage should be taken seriously; (2) when used as antitumor adjuvant in humans, the daily cimetidine dose is 100% to 150% of the standard dose for gastric ulcers.[35] If that standard were applied, the comparable equine dose would be 48 to 72 mg/kg/d.[40] The use of cimetidine, especially in combination with other therapies, deserves further examination. It should be noted that levamisole also is thought to inhibit Tregs and has been trialed extensively in human malignant melanoma, sometimes in combination with cimetidine.[41] Although levamisole has been used as an immunostimulant in other settings in the horse,[42,43] it does not seem to have been used for melanoma treatment.

Vaccines

Cancer vaccines are expected to activate the immune system as adjuvants and deliver antigens to T lymphocytes, resulting in the expansion of cytotoxic CD8-positive T cells to cause tumor regression. Human melanoma has been the target of numerous cancer vaccine efforts. By and large, the results have been disappointing.[35] The antigenic sources included in these vaccines were disialogangliosides, tumor cell lysates, allogeneic tumor cells, heat-shock proteins, and human leukocyte antigen–restricted peptides. Dendritic cell vaccines and mAbs are now at the forefront of vaccine approaches to human cancer and show early promise.[24,28] Several approaches to vaccination therapy have been tried in horses and are outlined in the following paragraphs.

Autologous whole-cell vaccines

Melanomas on 11 of 12 horses, given a whole-cell autogenous vaccine, were reported to have regressed, although the extent of tumor shrinkage and the duration of follow-ups are not reported.[44] These vaccines were produced from excised melanomas that were disassociated in collagenase, frozen, irradiated, and injected subcutaneously over regional lymph nodes weekly for 6 weeks, then every 6 weeks. A cell-wall–derived adjuvant was included for initial inoculations. Although the author has continued to make autogenous vaccine upon request over the decades since the original report, no updated efficacy information has been published. There is an anecdotal report of the use of freeze-thawed (irradiated?) cubes of melanoma tissue implanted subcutaneously as adjunctive therapy for gray horse melanoma, but results are unknown.[45] In another approach to whole-cell vaccination, melanomas are disassociated, put in tissue culture, transfected with the gene for the immunogenic protein *Streptococcus pyogenes* EMM55, irradiated, and administered to horses with melanoma in an attempt to break tolerance with a combination of self- and bacterial antigens (ImmuneFx vaccine; Morphogenesis, Tampa, FL). This vaccine, which may carry some risk of inducing purpura hemorrhagica in horses sensitized to *Streptococcus equi subsp. equi*, has been administered to horses for several years but efficacy data have not yet been reported.

Subunit vaccines
Disialogangliosides. Cells of neuroectodermal origin, including melanocytes, richly express the surface membrane disialogangliosides GD3 and GD2, making these antigens attractive targets for active or passive (ie, mAb) immunization against melanoma. Anti-GD2 and anti-GD3 mAbs enhanced multiple cytotoxicity mechanisms against canine melanoma cell lines.[28] Immunization with an adjuvanted GD3 vaccine generated robust antibody and cell-mediated responses in dogs and provided the rationale for ongoing trials in treatment of canine malignant melanoma.[46] This vaccine also has been used in a small number of horses with melanoma at the University of Florida. **Fig. 4** shows preliminary results from this trial. There was no significant change in size of 55 cutaneous melanoma masses in 14 horses followed-up for 1 to 2 years after a course of 4 intradermal GD3 vaccinations. Because there is no untreated control group and data ranges are wide, it is not yet clear whether or not there is an effect of vaccination on melanoma progression.

DNA vaccines
Tyrosinase. This vaccine (ONCEPT Canine melanoma vaccine, DNA; Boehringer Ingelheim Animal Health, USA) was the first anticancer vaccine to be approved by the United States Department of Agriculture. It is a bacterial plasmid vaccine encoding the *human tyrosinase* gene and is licensed for the treatment of dogs with oral malignant melanoma after locoregional control. Reports of efficacy have been contradictory and there is no consensus as to whether the vaccine should be recommended

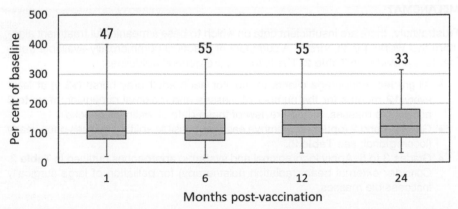

Fig. 4. Relative size of melanomas in 14 horses after GD3 vaccination. Horses were given 4 monthly doses of GD3 vaccine by intradermal injection. The maximal diameter of selected tumors on each of these horses were measured before (baseline), and at the intervals shown, after vaccination. Tukey boxes show median, first and third quartiles, and highest and lowest values.

Table 2	
Available treatments for locoregional and systemic treatment of gray horse melanoma	
Locoregional	**Systemic**
Removal	Immunomodulators
Surgery	Cimetidine[a]
Cryotherapy	± Levamisole[b]
CO_2 laser	
Chemotherapy	Vaccines
Cisplatin/Carboplatin	Human tyrosinase[c]
± Electroporation	Whole cell
± Hyperthermia	Whole cell/EMM55[d]

[a] Suggested dose −16 mg/kg by mouth 3 × daily for ≥3 mo.
[b] Suggested dose – 2.5 mg/kg by mouth 2 × weekly for ≥3 mo.
[c] ONCEPT (see text).
[d] ImmuneFx (see text).

routinely in canine malignant melanoma.[28] The ONCEPT vaccine is not licensed for horses but can be obtained for off label use by certified veterinary oncologists.[12] Pre-clinical investigation has shown that tyrosinase is constitutively expressed at high levels in equine melanomas and that the vaccine is safe and effective and generates robust antibody and cell-mediated responses against equine tyrosinase.[12] At least one clinical trial has been performed in horses with melanoma, and the vaccine is quite widely used in the United States. It was reported anecdotally that "most horses demonstrate[ed] tumor shrinkage after vaccination."[12] Quantitative efficacy data have not yet been reported, however. In a less encouraging study, which used a DNA minimal vector, inclusion of the human tyrosinase gene did not show any treatment advantage over transfection with the combination of IL-12 and IL-18.[32]

S pyogenes EMM55 protein. A gray horse with stage 5 melanoma was injected with 8 doses of DNA plasmid vaccine containing the S pyogenes emm55 gene.[47] There was substantial shrinkage of all tumors, including those that had not been injected.

IS THERE AN OVERALL STRATEGY FOR MANAGEMENT OF HORSES WITH MELANOMA?

Frustratingly, there are insufficient data on which to base a meaningful treatment algorithm that works for all horses. A summary of practical commercially available treatments is provided in **Table 2**. The following are general guidelines:

- All grades. Encourage clients to monitor each adult gray horse (>3 y) at least every 12 months for the number of masses and maximal dimension of up to 3 accessible masses. Include review of these data at wellness checks.
- Grades 1 and 2 (optional). Remove easily accessible solitary masses once yearly (locoregional; see **Table 2**).
- Grades 3 to 5. Apply locoregional and systemic approaches outlined in **Table 2**. Consider external beam radiation (teletherapy) for palliation of large surgically inaccessible masses.

REFERENCES

1. Pielberg GR, Golovko A, Sundstrom E, et al. A cis-acting regulatory mutation causes premature hair graying and susceptibility to melanoma in the horse. Nat Genet 2008;40:1004–9.

2. Sundstrom E, Imsland F, Mikko S, et al. Copy number expansion of the STX17 duplication in melanoma tissue from Grey horses. BMC Genomics 2012;13:365.
3. Curik I, Druml T, Seltenhammer M, et al. Complex inheritance of melanoma and pigmentation of coat and skin in Grey horses. PLoS Genet 2013;9:e1003248.
4. Teixeira RB, Rendahl AK, Anderson SM, et al. Coat color genotypes and risk and severity of melanoma in gray quarter horses. J Vet Intern Med 2013;27:1201–8.
5. Cichorek M, Wachulska M, Stasiewicz A, et al. Skin melanocytes: biology and development. Postepy Dermatol Alergol 2013;30:30–41.
6. Seltenhammer MH, Simhofer H, Scherzer S, et al. Equine melanoma in a population of 296 grey Lipizzaner horses. Equine Vet J 2003;35:153–7.
7. Fleury C, Berard F, Leblond A, et al. The study of cutaneous melanomas in Camargue-type gray-skinned horses (2): Epidemiological survey. Pigment Cell Res 2000;13:47–51.
8. Hofmanova B, Vostry L, Majzik I, et al. Characterization of greying, melanoma, and vitiligo quantitative inheritance in Old Kladruber horses. Czech J Anim Sci 2015;60:443–51.
9. Fleury C, Berard F, Balme B, et al. The study of cutaneous melanomas in Camargue-type gray-skinned horses (1): Clinical-pathological characterization. Pigment Cell Res 2000;13:39–46.
10. Comfort A. Coat-colour and longevity in thoroughbred mares. Nature 1958;182: 1531–2.
11. Cavalleri JMV, Malmann K, Steinig P, et al. Aetiology, clinical presentation and current treatment options of equine malignant melanoma - a review of the literature Abstracts. Pferdeheilkunde 2014;30:455–60.
12. Phillips JC, Lembcke LM. Equine melanocytic tumors. Vet Clin North Am Equine Pract 2013;29:673–87.
13. Johnson PJ. Dermatologic tumors (excluding sarcoids). Vet Clin North Am Equine Pract 1998;14:625–58.
14. Groom LM, Sullins KE. Surgical excision of large melanocytic tumours in grey horses: 38 cases (2001-2013). Equine Vet Educ 2018;30:438–43.
15. Theon AP. Intralesional and topical chemotherapy and immunotherapy. Vet Clin North Am Equine Pract 1998;14:659–71.
16. Theon AP, Wilson WD, Magdesian KG, et al. Long-term outcome associated with intratumoral chemotherapy with cisplatin for cutaneous tumors in equidae: 573 cases (1995-2004). J Am Vet Med Assoc 2007;230:1506–13.
17. Hewes CA, Sullins KE. Use of cisplatin-containing biodegradable beads for treatment of cutaneous neoplasia in equidae: 59 cases (2000-2004). J Am Vet Med Assoc 2006;229:1617–22.
18. Theon A. Cisplatin treatment of cutaneous tumors. In: Robinson N, editor. Current therapy in equine medicine. 4th edition. Philadelphia: WB Saunders; 1997. p. 372.
19. Campana LG, Testori A, Curatolo P, et al. Treatment efficacy with electrochemotherapy: a multi-institutional prospective observational study on 376 patients with superficial tumors. Eur J Surg Oncol 2016;42:1914–23.
20. Cemazar M, Tamzali Y, Sersa G, et al. Electrochemotherapy in veterinary oncology. J Vet Intern Med 2008;22:826–31.
21. Tamzali Y, Borde L, Rols MP, et al. Successful treatment of equine sarcoids with cisplatin electrochemotherapy: a retrospective study of 48 cases. Equine Vet J 2012;44:214–20.
22. Spugnini EP, D'Alterio GL, Dotsinsky I, et al. Electrochemotherapy for the treatment of multiple melanomas in a horse. J Equine Vet Sci 2011;31:430–3.

23. Scacco L, Bolaffio C, Romano A, et al. Adjuvant electrochemotherapy increases local control in a recurring equine anal melanoma. J Equine Vet Sci 2013;33: 637–9.

24. Mahmood J, Shukla HD, Soman S, et al. Immunotherapy, radiotherapy, and hyperthermia: a combined therapeutic approach in pancreatic cancer treatment. Cancer 2018;10 [pii:E469].

25. Henson FMD, Dobson JM. Use of radiation therapy in the treatment of equine neoplasia. Equine Vet Educ 2004;16:315–8.

26. Dixon J, Smith K, Perkins J, et al. Computed tomographic appearance of melanomas in the equine head: 13 cases. Vet Radiol Ultrasound 2016;57:246–52.

27. Bradley WM, Schilpp D, Khatibzadeh SM. Electronic brachytherapy used for the successful treatment of three different types of equine tumours. Equine Vet Educ 2017;29:293–8.

28. Almela RM, Anson A. A review of immunotherapeutic strategies in canine malignant melanoma. Vet Sci 2019;6 [pii:E15].

29. Dillman RO. Cancer immunotherapy. Cancer Biother Radiopharm 2011;26:1–64.

30. Heinzerling L, Feige K, Rieder S, et al. Tumor regression induced by intratumoral injection of DNA coding for human interleukin 12 into melanoma metastases in gray horses. J Mol Med 2001;78:692–702.

31. Muller JMV, Feige K, Wunderlin P, et al. Double-blind placebo-controlled study with interleukin-18 and interleukin-12-encoding plasmid DNA shows antitumor effect in metastatic melanoma in gray horses. J Immunother 2011;34:58–64.

32. Mahlmann K, Feige K, Juhls C, et al. Local and systemic effect of transfection-reagent formulated DNA vectors on equine melanoma. BMC Vet Res 2015;11.

33. Ribas A. Tumor immunotherapy directed at PD-1. N Engl J Med 2012;366: 2517–9.

34. Siegers CP, Andresen S, Keogh JP. Does cimetidine improve prospects for cancer patients?. A reappraisal of the evidence to date. Digestion 1999;60:415–21.

35. Lefranc F, Yeaton P, Brotchi J, et al. Cimetidine, an unexpected anti-tumor agent, and its potential for the treatment of glioblastoma. Int J Oncol 2006;28:1021–30.

36. Goetz TE, Ogilvie GK, Keegan KG, et al. Cimetidine for treatment of melanomas in 3 horses. J Am Vet Med Assoc 1990;196:449–52.

37. Goetz TE, Long MT. Treatment of melanomas in horses. Compend Contin Educ Vet 1993;15:608–10.

38. Hare JE, Staempfli HR. Cimetidine for the treatment of melanomas in horses - efficacy determined by client questionnaire. Equine Pract 1994;16:18–21.

39. Laus F, Cerquetella M, Paggi E, et al. Evaluation of cimetidine as a therapy for dermal melanomatosis in grey horse. Refu Vet 2010;65:48–52.

40. Smyth GB, Duran S, Ravis W, et al. Pharmacokinetic studies of cimetidine hydrochloride in adult horses. Equine Vet J 1990;22:48–50.

41. Molife R, Hancock BW. Adjuvant therapy of malignant melanoma. Crit Rev Oncol Hematol 2002;44:81–102.

42. Witonsky S, Buechner-Maxwell V, Santonastasto A, et al. Can levamisole upregulate the equine cell-mediated macrophage (M1) dendritic cell (DC1) T-helper 1 (CD4 Th1) T-cytotoxic (CD8) immune response in vitro? J Vet Intern Med 2019; 33:889–96.

43. Ellison SP, Lindsay DS. Decoquinate combined with levamisole reduce the clinical signs and serum SAG 1, 5, 6 antibodies in horses with suspected equine protozoal myeloencephalitis. Int J Appl Res Vet Med 2012;10:1–7.

44. Jeglum KA. Melanomas. In: Robinson NE, editor. Current therapy in equine medicine. 4th edition. Philadelphia: WB Saunders; 1997. p. 399–400.

45. Metcalfe LVA, O'Brien PJ, Papakonstantinou S, et al. Malignant melanoma in a grey horse: case presentation and review of equine melanoma treatment options. Ir Vet J 2013;66:22.
46. Milner RJ, Salute M, Crawford C, et al. The immune response to disialoganglioside GD3 vaccination in normal dogs: a melanoma surface antigen vaccine. Vet Immunol Immunopathol 2006;114:273–84.
47. Brown EL, Ramiya VK, Wright CA, et al. Treatment of metastatic equine melanoma with a plasmid DNA vaccine encoding Streptococcus pyogenes EMM55 protein. J Equine Vet Sci 2014;34:704–8.

Diagnostic Testing for Equine Endocrine Diseases
Confirmation Versus Confusion

Dianne McFarlane, DVM, PhD

KEYWORDS

- Equine pituitary pars intermedia dysfunction • Equine metabolic syndrome • ACTH
- Insulin

KEY POINTS

- No diagnostic tests should be interpreted without consideration of signalment, history, and specific clinical signs of disease.
- Measurement of hormones, both baseline or after stimulation, is affected by many other factors, including concurrent illness, season, thriftiness, color, breed, and diet.
- Any diagnostic test is only as good as the assay measuring the hormone.
- Reference intervals are only valid for a specific method and assay. Breed-specific reference intervals are needed.

Although once a fairly obscure field, equine endocrinology now holds great interest to the horse-owning public. The 2 common endocrine syndromes, pituitary pars intermedia dysfunction (PPID) and equine metabolic syndrome (EMS), are each frequently featured in horse industry news outlets. In addition, the availability of highly marketed pharmaceuticals has contributed to heightened awareness of these conditions by veterinarians and clients alike. As awareness of equine endocrine diseases has grown, more owners are requesting their horses be tested, often in the absence of convincing clinical signs supportive of disease. Unfortunately, the current diagnostic tests are poor at predicting endocrine disease when only minimal or nonspecific clinical signs are present.

Equine endocrinology is a field that has undergone numerous transformations, with its share of incorrect conclusions along the way. For example, historically it was

Disclosure Statement: Dr D. McFarlane has no conflict of interest. She has participated in the Equine Endocrinology Group that provides recommendations on diagnostic testing for PPID that is distributed by Boehringer Ingelheim (BI) in marketing handouts and in the Equine Endocrine Summit (a small group scientific meeting), both of which have been supported by BI.
Department of Physiological Sciences, Center for Veterinary Health Sciences, Oklahoma State University, 264 McElroy Hall, CVHS-OSU, Stillwater, OK 74078, USA
E-mail address: diannem@okstate.edu

thought that hypothyroidism was a common equine disease and the mechanism behind obesity-associated laminitis in horses. Many horses were prescribed lifelong treatment with levothyroxine as a result. Later, the role of dysfunctional thyroid glands in obesity-related laminitis was challenged, and the concept that hyperinsulinemia was responsible for inciting endocrinopathic laminitis was introduced.[1] Along with a new understanding of the mechanism of endocrinopathic laminitis came a new name for this condition, equine metabolic syndrome (EMS).[2] The definition of EMS has evolved since the term was first introduced in 2002, and changes in diagnostic and treatment approaches have followed.[2]

The understanding of equine PPID has also undergone many shifts in the past several decades. Once thought to be an uncommon condition, PPID affects 20% to 30% of the geriatric horse population.[3–5] Clinical signs attributed to PPID have often been based on poorly defined cases, and as a result, are inaccurate. Originally called "equine Cushing disease," the condition was thought to be similar to human and canine Cushing disease. Pituitary-dependent hyperadrenocorticism was considered to be the mechanistic cause, despite an inability to demonstrate high-serum cortisol concentrations or enlarged adrenal glands in most equine cases.[6–8] These misconceptions pervaded the veterinary literature for several decades.

Over the years, many diagnostic tests have been suggested that ultimately were proven to be poor discriminators of disease. Problems from "interference" due to physiologic endocrine activity, from overgeneralizing data collected in a small number of nonrepresentative animals, poor case definition, to a lack of a gold standard, plagued validation studies.

This article is not intended to serve as an exhaustive review of equine endocrine disease or testing strategies. Several comprehensive reviews have been recently published.[9–12] Rather, it discusses areas in the field of equine endocrine disease diagnosis that need further consideration due to common misconceptions or misuse of the current recommendations. In addition, suggestions for future directions for enhanced diagnostic capabilities in equine endocrinology are included.

ASSAY MATTERS

It is important that the diagnostic tests used to identify cases have been appropriately validated and that guidelines for interpretation of results be broadly applicable and accurate. *A well-accepted but often overlooked fact is that reference intervals are only valid for the specific assay and methodology for which they were established.* There are numerous reports comparing the performance of radioimmunoassays, enzyme-linked immunosorbent assays (ELISAs), chemiluminescent immunoassay, and immunofluorescent assays for measuring adrenocorticotropic hormone (ACTH), insulin, and other hormones; all show bias or lack of agreement among the assays, with a high percentage of discordant samples.[13–18] Therefore, results among assays are not interchangeable, and reference intervals provided by laboratories or diagnostic guidelines are only relevant if the samples are run using the same methodology. When monitoring patients over time, the same method of hormone measurement must be used if current and previous results are to be compared.

It is also important to understand the limitations and specificity of the assay used. Most assays used to measure equine hormones are designed for use in other species, most commonly human-specific assays. Validation for use with equine samples is required, and details of the validation should be publicly available. Unfortunately, often the validation process performed is not ideal. This failure to appropriately valid assays may be the consequence of an absence of an unequivocal method (a "gold standard") or a lack of available species-specific reagents. Some assays cross-react with other similar molecules. For example, the chemiluminescent immunoassay (Immulite) for ACTH has 13% to 15% cross-reactivity with corticotropin-like intermediate lobe peptide (CLIP) when human plasma is the test sample (Immulite 1000 ACTH Product literature; Siemens Medical Solutions USA, Inc. Malvern, PA). Cross-reactivity with CLIP likely also occurs in horses.[18] Thus, fall samples measured by chemiluminescent immunoassay will report higher ACTHs compared with the same samples measured by other methods with minimal cross-reactivity. The cross-reactivity with CLIP does not make this assay inappropriate for PPID; it is, however, an important consideration when interpreting results.

There are limited methods for measuring equine insulin concentration, and the available tests show poor assay performance.[15] Using liquid chromatography–mass spectrometry (LC-MS) as the unequivocal measure of insulin concentration, 6 insulin assays were compared.[15] Of the 6 tested, 2 had adequate assay characteristics (precision, accuracy, and specificity) to be valid for measuring equine insulin. Of those, only 1 correlated to the absolute insulin concentration determined by LC-MS, and it identified only 25% to 50% of the actual insulin in the sample. This assay is no longer available.

Recent evaluation of the chemiluminescent immunoassay revealed suitable performance characteristics with lower results compared with those obtained by radioimmunoassay or ELISA.[19] Evaluations of the ability of the chemiluminescent immunoassay or currently available radioimmunoassays to identify equine insulin using the unequivocal method of LC-MS as a reference have not been reported.

EQUINE PITUITARY PARS INTERMEDIA DYSFUNCTION

Many diagnostic tests for PPID have come and gone out of favor over the years. Today, the most frequently used test in practice is endogenous plasma ACTH concentration, and the test considered to be most discriminating is the thyrotropin-releasing hormone (TRH) stimulation assay.[20,21] The overnight dexamethasone suppression test (DST), although no longer commonly used, is still considered an appropriate albeit less sensitive diagnostic test. All of the current tests have their strengths and weaknesses; understanding how to best use and interpret the available tests will aid in a better likelihood of reaching an accurate diagnosis.

The Physiology and Pathophysiology

PPID is the result of a loss of inhibitory regulation of the melanotropes of the pars intermedia lobe of the pituitary resulting in increased release of POMC peptides, α-MSH, ACTH, β-endorphin, and CLIP along with many less-defined small peptides.[22,23] Loss of inhibitory regulation is the result of loss of hypothalamic dopaminergic neurons, which serve to provide tonic inhibition to the pars intermedia.[24] The pars intermedia has several known roles in other species, including regulation of seasonal change in metabolism, appetite, and hair coat, presumably to prepare animals for the challenges of winter.[25–27] It provides powerful anti-inflammatory hormones in response to cytokine stimulation.[28] Although much remains unknown, available data suggest similar functions in horses.[29,30] Removal of dopaminergic innervation, as occurs with PPID, results in an exaggerated seasonal increase in pars intermedia hormones.[31]

Interpreting the results of the PPID diagnostic tests is complicated by the difficulty in separating an appropriate physiologic response of the pituitary from an inappropriate, dysregulated state. As discussed above, PPID is a disease in which dopaminergic inhibition is lost. However, all current diagnostic tests for PPID work by measuring pars intermedia activity (they directly or indirectly assess ACTH release) rather than dopaminergic neuronal activity. None are able to characterize whether ACTH is of pars intermedia or pars distalis origin.

Why Is This a Problem?

ACTH release can be upregulated without loss of dopaminergic neuronal function. Horses in extremely poor condition and those with chronic or acute disease may exhibit an increase in plasma ACTH without reducing dopaminergic activity.[32] Significant variability exists among horses in the magnitude of hormonal response to both season and inflammation. Gray horses often have a greater fall increase in proopiomelanocortin (POMC) peptides compared with other colored horses.[33] Thrifty breeds of ponies have been shown to have dramatic increases in ACTH activity in the fall.[33,34] In other species, dopaminergic tone is related to metabolism, appetite, and obesity.[35,36] It is possible that genetically thrifty animals have less dopaminergic tone (ie, neurons) than nonthrifty breeds to promote a stronger seasonal response of the pars intermedia, thus creating a heightened thrifty response. These genetic differences are likely advantageous to the younger animal needing to survive in harsh winter environments but may predispose to PPID later in life, because the number of functioning dopaminergic neurons are known to decrease with age.[37,38]

Dopaminergic tone can also be influenced by environmental factors in addition to genetics. Antenatal exposure to glucocorticoids or stress has been shown to decrease the number of functional dopaminergic neurons.[39,40] In intrauterine growth-restricted children, variation in dopamine signaling is associated with changes in eating behavior.[41] It is possible that in horses predisposition to PPID is influenced by the initial population density of dopaminergic neurons, which is determined by a combination of breed and environmental factors.

In summary, breed variation may contribute to differences in dopaminergic tone as a function of thriftiness and other phenotypes (eg, color), which must be considered when interpreting diagnostic test results. A large seasonal increase in plasma ACTH concentration, endogenous or stimulated, may be normal. It should not automatically be assumed that a horse has PPID, especially if that horse is young and lacks clinical signs. Although low-dopaminergic tone and a strong seasonal pars intermedia response may be advantageous (and normal) in the younger thrifty animal, it may also present a risk factor for PPID later in life. Therefore, a finding of a strong ACTH seasonal response in a younger horse is cause to monitor that animal as it ages. Ideally, tests for PPID will be developed that directly assess the ability of the periventricular dopaminergic neurons to respond appropriately to stimulation, by releasing dopamine.

Tests for Pituitary Pars Intermedia Dysfunction Measuring Adrenocorticotropic Hormone

Endogenous plasma ACTH can be produced by 2 types of pituitary cells, corticotropes of the pars distalis and melanotropes of the pars intermedia. An increase in plasma concentration may occur due to stimulation of either cell type; current diagnostic tests cannot differentiate these 2 events. Tests also cannot separate an appropriate response to an environmental event from a pathologic, unregulated release of ACTH. Therefore, it is essential that the interpretation of plasma ACTH concentration only be made in light of the history, signalment, season of sample collection, and clinical findings of the patient.

ACTH is a cleavage product from the larger polypeptide, POMC. In the non-fall season, nearly all ACTH in healthy horses is from the pars distalis and is posttranslationally modified such that it is bioactive. In horses with PPID or during the fall, the increase in ACTH is due to pars intermedia hormone production. Most of the pars intermedia ACTH is post-translationally modified to a nonbioactive form.[42,43] Therefore, although current tests do not differentiate ACTH from the 2 pituitary cell types, development of more specific tests is feasible based on differences in ACTH structure or function (bioactivity).

Plasma ACTH concentration increases in horses with PPID. However, it may also increase with chronic and acute disease, malnutrition, and other stressors. *Consequently, detection of a high ACTH concentration does not confirm the diagnosis of PPID.* Plasma ACTH concentration is affected by breed, age, coat color, thriftiness, diet, health status, time of year, and location of residence.[32–34,44–46] ACTH is released from the pituitary in a pulsatile fashion with as much as a 2-fold difference in plasma concentrations over a 1-hour collection period in normal horses, suggesting significant intrahorse variation may be normal.[47] In contrast, other studies with less frequent sample collection failed to demonstrate ultradian rhythm, and collection of paired sampling did not improve sensitivity or specificity of the test.[48,49] Attempts to calculate the sensitivity and specificity of plasma ACTH concentration in diagnosis of PPID are thwarted by the absence of a gold-standard diagnostic test. As a result, a diagnosis of PPID must be based on more than just a high endogenous plasma ACTH concentration.

Thyrotropin-releasing hormone stimulation test

The TRH stimulation test is a dynamic diagnostic test that measures the magnitude of plasma ACTH increase following intravenous administration of the natural pituitary releasing factor, TRH.[50] The primary benefit of the dynamic test is the ability to standardize the stimulus and synchronize the response. Samples in the TRH stimulation test are collected before and 10 minutes after TRH administration.[21] The magnitude of the increase in plasma ACTH at 10 minutes after stimulation is an indication of the hormone content stored in the pars intermedia melanotropes and pars distalis corticotropes.[51] Because of the large variability in TRH response among horses in the fall, seasonal reference intervals are unlikely to be useful in the diagnosis of PPID. Age, color, breed, thriftiness, and diet all may have an influence on magnitude of ACTH response in the fall. Despite this, there may be value in performing the TRH stimulation test in the fall. Horses showing minimal ACTH response to TRH in the fall have a very strong probability of *not* having PPID, making the test useful to rule out, not rule in, PPID. Other concerns regarding interpretation of TRH stimulation test results include the lack of data on the effect of concurrent disease on test response or timing of sample collection. In other species ACTH is removed primarily through renal excretion, with a half-life under 1 minute.[52] The effect of imprecise timing of the post-TRH 10-minute sample or concurrent renal disease on test results has not been adequately assessed.

Overnight Dexamethasone Suppression Test

In 1994, Dybdal and colleagues[53] suggested the DST had 100% sensitivity and specificity, and the DST became the standard for PPID diagnosis for the next decade. Later, it became clear that the performance of the DST was less discriminating than originally suggested. Furthermore, owner concern regarding the safety of dexamethasone in horses that might be predisposed to laminitis resulted in many opting not to test their horses.

Test mechanism

In healthy horses, administration of dexamethasone suppresses adrenal cortisol release by inhibiting corticotrope-derived ACTH and hypothalamic corticotropin-releasing hormone secretion. Glucocorticoids do not inhibit ACTH production by pars intermedia melanotropes.

Current recommended interpretation

When the test is performed in the non-fall season, serum cortisol greater than 1 μg/dL at 19 hours after dexamethasone administration is considered a failure to suppress and consistent with PPID.[53] This cutoff was determined using a population of end-stage PPID cases compared with clinically healthy age-matched horses. Disease state was confirmed at postmortem.[53] Ideally, one should validate a diagnostic test in a random, representative population and compare the results with a gold standard. Pre-selection of animals as diseased or normal will overestimate the sensitivity and specificity of the test, as occurred with the DST.

Limitations

The DST has a low sensitivity and high specificity. Using the diagnostic cutoff of cortisol less than 1 μg/dL at 19 hours after dexamethasone administration, only horses with late-stage PPID fail to suppress.[54] False negatives are common in early cases of PPID. Repeat testing is often necessary to diagnose early cases. False positives may occur when the test is performed in the fall, and seasonally, specific reference intervals have not been established. However, horses that fully suppress to less than 0.2 μg/dL (typical limit of detection of the assay) in the fall are very likely NOT to have PPID.

Maximizing dexamethasone suppression test potential

Several changes can be made to the DST to enhance its predictive value. Typically, horses with serum cortisol greater than 1 μg/dL at 19 hours after dexamethasone administration are considered to have PPID. However, horses with early PPID may have post-dexamethasone cortisol concentrations in the moderate (0.5–1 μg/dL) range. Further research is needed to redefine the best diagnostic cutoffs. Early cases of PPID may be better identified by collecting the second sample at 24 rather than 19 hours after dexamethasone administration, because some horses with early disease will suppress initially and then escape, whereas normal horses will remain suppressed.[53] One of the limitations of this test, and perhaps why it fails to identify early cases, is that ACTH produced in the pars intermedia is posttranslationally modified such that it is often not bioactive: it does not stimulate adrenal release of cortisol.[42,43] Development of an assay that differentiates the various structural forms of ACTH (and thus the origin of ACTH) could strengthen the performance of the DST as well as other diagnostic tests for PPID.

Other Pituitary Pars Intermedia Dysfunction Tests Measuring Cortisol

Multiple studies have agreed that measurement of serum cortisol is not useful in the diagnosis of PPID.[8,53,54] Loss of cortisol diurnal rhythm has been proposed as a test for PPID[55]; however, although circadian rhythm of cortisol is disrupted in horses with PPID, it is also often disrupted in many other disease conditions and in otherwise healthy horses. In a small study of 46 healthy horses, the authors found 70% would have been falsely diagnosed as having PPID using diurnal cortisol change. Cortisol release following TRH administration also has an inadequate performance to be clinically useful.[51] ACTH stimulation was once used in the diagnosis of PPID and continues to be the test of choice to characterize PPID-associated adrenal hyperplasia.[53] However, nearly two-thirds of horses with PPID do not have adrenal hyperplasia and would test as false negatives.[6,7]

Recently, measurement of free cortisol was found to increase in horses with PPID, EMS, obesity, and hyperinsulinemia.[8] It is not clear whether a high free cortisol is useful in identifying specific endocrine disorders or how concurrent diseases might affect the results.

EQUINE METABOLIC SYNDROME

EMS is a list of clinical signs or pathologic conditions that, if present, increase risk of endocrinopathic laminitis.[56] Among these risk factors, insulin dysregulation is the strongest predictor of laminitis.

Insulin-glucose regulation is complex, and different parts of the insulin-glucose regulatory pathway may be altered in horses that have insulin dysregulation. Consequently, not all horses with insulin dysregulation will respond similarly to a specific diagnostic test.

The specificity of individual diagnostic tests in assessing insulin-glucose regulation is illustrated by a series of studies investigating metformin efficacy. Initial studies considered the ability of metformin to improve insulin sensitivity in horses using a frequently sampled intravenous glucose tolerance test.[57] No improvement was observed. Later work used an oral glucose test and demonstrated a highly significant reduction in both glucose and insulin concentration.[58] Pharmacokinetic studies suggest metformin is not well absorbed when given orally to horses.[59] However, in other species, metformin can elicit a local gastrointestinal effect, reducing small intestinal glucose absorption and subsequent pancreatic insulin release. A local gastrointestinal effect would only be appreciated with an oral glucose challenge test, not an intravenous glucose challenge. Although a local effect of metformin in the horse has not been indisputably demonstrated, this explanation fits all the available equine data.

The story of metformin in horses serves as an example of how results from the various diagnostics tests are not interchangeable, and no one diagnostic test is ideal for all cases. Some horses and ponies with EMS have a more profound tissue insulin resistance, whereas others have a more exaggerated glucose-stimulated insulin release. Both pathways lead to hyperinsulinemia and thus increased risk of endocrinopathic laminitis.

Baseline Testing

Equine serum insulin concentration
Measurement of serum insulin concentration as a diagnostic test for insulin resistance is a noninvasive, technically easy method. However, false negative results are extremely common.[21] Guidelines suggest normal serum insulin concentration is less than 20 μU/mL; however, for some breeds, normal serum insulin concentration is lower.[60] Opinions on the best type of resting sample (fasted, fed, or feed restricted) change frequently and continue to be debated. Current recommendations suggest withholding grain but allowing availability to hay or pasture when testing.

Dynamic Testing

Oral sugar or glucose tests
To reduce the high false negative rate, a dynamic test is suggested. Postprandial insulin release may be assessed using an oral sugar test or an in-feed oral glucose test. The oral sugar test provides the horse a sugar bolus in the form of Karo syrup administered via dose syringe.[61] The in-feed oral glucose test provides a sugar bolus in the form of dextrose powder in a nonglycemic feed such as chaff.[62] Both evaluate glucose absorption and postprandial insulin release. Debates regarding these tests center primarily on the optimal dose of sugar and degree of fasting. Significant breed differences occur, suggesting multiple reference intervals are needed.[60]

Intravenous insulin tolerance tests

To assess tissue-level insulin sensitivity, an insulin tolerance test is recommended. The 2-step insulin response test is the simplest to perform in practice, but has the potential to induce clinical hypoglycemia if the horse is not insulin resistant.[63] The 2-step insulin response test measures glucose response at 30 minutes, making it both inexpensive and convenient, providing immediate stall-side results. Fasting is not recommended. The combined intravenous glucose-insulin tolerance test avoids the risk of hypoglycemia but is a more labor intensive alternative.[64]

REACHING A CORRECT DIAGNOSIS: WHY IS IT SO COMPLICATED?

Diagnosis of endocrine disease requires a holistic approach incorporating history, signalment, and clinical examination findings together with diagnostic test results. Because the function of the endocrine system is to maintain homeostasis, change in environment or animal health will alter hormone response. Failing to consider the horse as a whole and treating based on laboratory test results have caused many animals to receive lifelong drug treatment unnecessarily. Several factors may complicate diagnosis of endocrine disease in the horse.

Slowly Progressive, Insidious Diseases

The slow progression from disease onset to end-stage disease has implications in diagnostic testing and test validation. Cases of early endocrine disease will have unique clinical and pathologic characteristics compared with late disease. For example, early in disease, loss of dopaminergic inhibition may increase prolactin secretion. Late in disease, compression of the lactotrophs in the pars distalis might cause a decrease in prolactin. Failure to stratify horses by disease stage could lead to the conclusion that prolactin concentration is not altered in horses with PPID when in fact prolactin was affected both early and late in disease. This theoretic example illustrates the importance of considering not just if the horse has an endocrine disease but also where they fall on a chronicity timeline when considering diagnostic results.

Concurrent Endocrine Diseases

Another common complexity when evaluating horses for endocrine disease is that clinical endocrine syndromes may occur alone or in combination, and each presentation will have its own unique appearance. One will encounter horses with PPID alone, intermedia dysfunction (ID) (EMS) alone, or PPID and ID. PPID horses with normal insulin regulation do not appear to be at increased risk of laminitis or obesity. Conversely, horses with PPID and ID appear to be at greater risk of hyperinsulinemia and laminitis than ID alone. One-third of the horses with PPID will also have adrenal hyperplasia. It is unclear if these horses have unique clinical signs or response to treatment. A small number of horses with PPID, ID or PPID, and ID will go on to develop diabetes mellitus. If one fails to assess glucose and insulin concurrently, this may be overlooked, and management of the patient will likely be inappropriate.

Multiple Pathways Leading to the Same Endpoint

There are likely multiple causes for both PPID and EMS that ultimately converge into similar end-stage clinical signs. In PPID, many events may cause dopaminergic neurodegeneration, such as toxins, oxidative stress, metabolic derangements, mitochondrial dysfunction, excessive dopamine exposure, or genetic predisposition to overexpress proteins that misfold. Early in disease, each of these underlying disease mechanisms may be associated with unique biomarkers and response to diagnostic tests. However, regardless of the initiating event, once the dopaminergic neurons are no longer able to tonically inhibit the pars intermedia, the end-stage syndrome will be indistinguishable: excessive release of pars intermedia hormones with the associated clinical signs.

EMS also has different causes. Hyperinsulinemia, the key abnormality in EMS, can result from either tissue level insulin resistance or excessive postprandial insulin release. Multiple risk factors, such as obesity, inflammation, toxins, breed, and diet, initiate different pathologic events that all ultimately cause insulin dysregulation and increased risk of laminitis. Interpretation of diagnostic test results for EMS must consider cause, because a test of insulin-sensitive tissue response will not identify EMS horses with insulin dysregulation because of excessive postprandial pancreatic insulin release.

Physiologic Responses Overlap with Pathologic Responses

Glands have jobs; they release hormones as needed to maintain homeostasis. They respond to physiologic events, such as season or diet, and pathologic events, such as illness, debilitation, or stress. When testing endocrine function rather than asking "is hormone production increased (with or without stimulation)?," it would be ideal to ask "can the system respond appropriately to positive and negative signals at multiple levels of the axis?"

REFERENCES

1. Patterson-Kane JC, Karikoski NP, McGowan CM. Paradigm shifts in understanding equine laminitis. Vet J 2018;231:33–40.
2. Johnson PJ. The equine metabolic syndrome peripheral Cushing's syndrome. Vet Clin North Am Equine Pract 2002;18:271–93.
3. McGowan TW, Pinchbeck GP, McGowan CM. Prevalence, risk factors and clinical signs predictive for equine pituitary pars intermedia dysfunction in aged horses. Equine Vet J 2013;45:74–9.
4. Brosnahan MM, Paradis MR. Assessment if clinical characteristics, management practices, and activities of geriatric horses. J Am Vet Med Assoc 2003;223: 99–103.
5. Ireland JL, McGowan CM. Epidemiology of pituitary pars intermedia dysfunction: a systematic literature review of clinical presentation, disease prevalence and risk factors. Vet J 2018;235:22–3.
6. Glover CM, Miller LM, Dybdal NO, et al. Extrapituitary and pituitary findings in horses with pituitary pars intermedia dysfunction: a retrospective study. J Equine Vet Sci 2009;29:146–53.
7. Boujon CE, Bestetti GE, Meier HP, et al. Equine pituitary adenoma: a functional and morphological study. J Comp Pathol 1993;109:163–78.
8. Hart KA, Wochele DM, Norton NA. Effect of age, season, body condition, and endocrine status on serum free cortisol fraction and insulin concentration in horses. J Vet Intern Med 2016;30:653–63.
9. Durham AE. Endocrine disease in aged horses. Vet Clin North Am Equine Pract 2016;32:301–15.
10. Spelta CW. Equine pituitary pars intermedia dysfunction: current perspectives on diagnosis and management. Vet Med (Auckl) 2015;6:293–300.
11. Morgan R, Keen J, McGowan CM. Equine metabolic syndrome. Vet Rec 2015; 177:179.

12. Bertin FR. The diagnosis of equine insulin dysregulation. Equine Vet J 2017;49: 570–6.
13. Banse HE, McCann J, Yang F, et al. Comparison of two methods for measurement of equine insulin. J Vet Diagn Invest 2014;26:527–30.
14. Borer-Weir KE, Bailey SR, Mendies-Gow NJ, et al. Evaluation of commercially available radioimmunoassay and species specific ELISAs for measurement of high concentrations of insulin in equine serum. Am J Vet Res 2012;73:1596–602.
15. Tinworth KD, Wynn PC, Boston RC, et al. Evaluation of commercially available assays for the measurement of equine insulin. Domest Anim Endocrinol 2011;41: 81–90.
16. Banse HE, Schultz N, McCue M, et al. Comparison of two methods for measurement of equine adrenocorticotropin. J Vet Diagn Invest 2018;30:233–7.
17. Irvine KL, Burt K, Hill AJ, et al. Initial analytic quality assessment and method comparison of an immunoassay for adrenocorticotropic hormone measurement in equine samples. Vet Clin Pathol 2016;45:154–63.
18. Knowles EJ, Moreton-Clack MC, Shae S, et al. Plasma adrenocorticotropic hormone (ACTH) concentrations in ponies measured by two different assays suggests seasonal cross-reactivity or interference. Equine Vet J 2018;50:672–7.
19. Carslake HB, Pinchbeck GL, McGowan CM. Evaluation of a chemiluminescent immunoassay for measurement of equine insulin. J Vet Intern Med 2017;31: 568–74.
20. Carmalt JL, Waldner CL, Allen AL. Equine pituitary pars intermedia dysfunction: an international survey of veterinarians' approach to diagnosis, management, and estimated prevalence. Can J Vet Res 2017;81:261–9.
21. Available at: https://sites.tufts.edu/equineendogroup/files/2017/11/2017-EEG-Recommendations-PPID.pdf. Accessed April 4, 2019.
22. McFarlane D. Pathophysiology and clinical features of pituitary pars intermedia dysfunction. Equine Vet Educ 2014;26:592–8.
23. McFarlane D. Equine pituitary pars intermedia dysfunction. Vet Clin North Am Equine Pract 2011;27:93–113.
24. McFarlane D, Dybdal N, Donaldson MT, et al. Nitration and increased alpha synuclein expression associated with dopaminergic neurodegeneration in equine pituitary pars intermedia dysfunction. J Neuroendocrinol 2005;17:73–80.
25. Lincoln GA, Rhind SM, Pompolo S, et al. Hypothalamic control of photoperiod-induced cycles in food intake, body weight, and metabolic hormones in rams. Am J Physiol Regul Integr Comp Physiol 2001;281:R76–90.
26. Schuhler S, Ebling FJ. Role of melanocortin in the long-term regulation of energy balance: lessons from a seasonal model. Peptides 2006;27:301–9.
27. Niklowitz F, Hoffmann K. Pineal and pituitary involvement in the photoperiodic regulation of body weight, coat color and testicular size of the Djungarian Hamster, Phodopus sungorus. Biol Reprod 1988;39:489–98.
28. Singh M, Mukhopadhyay K. Alpha-melanocyte stimulating hormone: an emerging anti-inflammatory antimicrobial peptide. Biomed Res Int 2014;2014:874610.
29. McFarlane D, Hill K, Anton J. Neutrophil function in healthy aged horses and horses with pituitary dysfunction. Vet Immunol Immunopathol 2015;165:99–106.
30. McFarlane D, Holbrook TC. Cytokine dysregulation in aged horses and horses with pituitary pars intermedia dysfunction. J Vet Intern Med 2008;22:436–42.
31. Copas VE, Durham AE. Circannual variation in plasma adrenocorticotropic hormone concentrations in the UK in normal horses and ponies, and those with pituitary pars intermedia dysfunction. Equine Vet J 2012;44:440–3.

32. Stewart AJ, Hacket E, Towns TJ, et al. Cortisol and ACTH concentrations in hospitalized horses. In: 40th Bain Fallon Memorial Lectures, Equine Veterinarians Australia Annual Conference, Sydney, Australia, July 15-18, 2019.

33. Durham A, Shreeve H. Horse factors influencing the seasonal increase in plasma ACTH secretion. In: Dorothy Russell Havemeyer Foundation International Equine Endocrinology Summit. 2017 36-37. Available at: https://sites.tufts.edu/equineendogroup/files/2017/01/2017-Equine-Endocrinology-Summit-D-Russell-Havemeyer-Foundation.pdf. Accessed April 4, 2019.

34. Fredrick J, McFarlane D. ACTH release following TRH stimulation in thrifty horses compared to metabolically normal horses. J Vet Intern Med 2014;28:1104.

35. Guo J, Simmons WK, Herscovitch P, et al. Striatal dopamine D2-like receptor correlation patterns with human obesity and opportunistic eating behavior. Mol Psychiatry 2014;19:1078–84.

36. Rubi B, Maechler P. New roles for peripheral dopamine on metabolic control and tumor growth: let's seek the balance. Endocrinology 2010;151:5570–81.

37. McGeer P, Itagaki S, Akiyama H, et al. Rate of cell death in Parkinson's disease indicates active neuropathological process. Ann Neurol 1988;24:574–6.

38. Fernley JM, Lees AJ. Ageing and Parkinson's disease: substantia nigra regional selectivity. Brain 1991;114:2283–301.

39. Leão P, Sousa JC, Oliveira M, et al. Programming effects of antenatal dexamethasone in the developing mesolimbic pathways. Synapse 2007;61:40–9.

40. Berger MA, Barros VG, Sarchi MI, et al. Long-term effects of prenatal stress on dopamine and glutamate receptors in adult rat brain. Neurochem Res 2002;27:1525–33.

41. Silveira PP, Pokhvisneva I, Gaudreau H, et al. Fetal growth interacts with multilocus genetic score reflecting dopamine signaling capacity to predict spontaneous sugar intake in children. Appetite 2018;120:596–601.

42. Cordero M, Scrauner B, McFarlane D. Bioactivity of plasma ACTH from PPID-affected horses compared to normal horses. J Vet Intern Med 2011;25:664.

43. Orth DN, Nicholson WE. Bioactive and immunoreactive adrenocorticotropin in normal equine pituitary and in pituitary tumors of horses with Cushing's disease. Endocrinology 1982;111:559–63.

44. Jacob SI, Geor RJ, Weber PS, et al. Effect of dietary carbohydrates and time of year on ACTH and cortisol concentrations in adult and aged horses. Domest Anim Endocrinol 2018;63:15–22.

45. Secombe CJ, Tan RHH, Perara DI, et al. The effect of geographic location on circannual adrenocorticotropic hormone plasma concentration in horses in Australia. J Vet Intern Med 2017;31:1533–40.

46. McFarlane D, Paradis MR, Zimmel D, et al. The effect of geographic location, breed and pituitary dysfunction on seasonal adrenocorticotropin and a-melanocyte stimulating hormone plasma concentration in horses. J Vet Intern Med 2011;25:872–81.

47. Carmalt JL, Duke-Novakovski T, Schott HC III, et al. Effects of anesthesia with isoflurane on plasma concentrations of adrenocorticotropic hormone in samples obtained from the cavernous sinus and jugular vein of horses. Am J Vet Res 2016;77:730–7.

48. Rendle DI, Litchfield E, Heller J, et al. Investigation of rhythms of secretion and repeatability of plasma adrenocorticotropic hormone concentrations in healthy horses and horses with pituitary pars intermedia dysfunction. Equine Vet J 2014;46:113–7.

49. Rendle DI, Duz M, Beech J, et al. Investigation of single and paired measurements of adrenocorticotropic hormone for the diagnosis of pituitary pars intermedia dysfunction in horses. J Vet Intern Med 2015;29:355–61.

50. Beech J, Boston R, Lindborg S, et al. Adrenocorticotropin concentration following administration of thyrotropin-releasing hormone in healthy horses and those with pituitary pars intermedia dysfunction and pituitary gland hyperplasia. J Am Vet Med Assoc 2007;231:417–26.

51. McFarlane D, Beech J, Cribb A. Alpha-melanocyte stimulating hormone release in response to thyrotropin releasing hormone in healthy horses, horses with pituitary pars intermedia dysfunction and equine pars intermedia explants. Domest Anim Endocrinol 2006;30:276–88.

52. Jones CT, Luther E, Ritchie JWK, et al. The clearance of ACTH from the plasma of adult and fetal sheep. Endocrinology 1975;96:231–4.

53. Dybdal NO, Hargreaves KM, Madigan JE, et al. Diagnostic testing for pituitary pars intermedia dysfunction in horses. J Am Vet Med Assoc 1994;204:627–32.

54. McFarlane D, Breshears MA, Cordero M, et al. Comparison of plasma ACTH concentration, plasma α-MSH concentration, and overnight dexamethasone suppression test for diagnosis of PPID. J Vet Intern Med 2012;30:253.

55. Douglas R. Circadian cortisol rhythmicity and equine Cushing's-like disease. J Equine Vet Sci 1999;19:684–753.

56. Frank N, Geor RJ, Bailey SR, et al. Equine metabolic syndrome. J Vet Intern Med 2010;24:467–75.

57. Tinworth KD, Boston RC, Harris PA, et al. The effect of oral metformin on insulin sensitivity in insulin-resistant ponies. Vet J 2012;191:79–84.

58. Rendle DI, Rutledge F, Hughes KJ, et al. Effects of metformin hydrochloride on blood glucose and insulin responses to oral dextrose in horses. Equine Vet J 2013;45:751–4.

59. Tinworth KD, Edwards S, Noble GK, et al. Pharmacokinetics of metformin after enteral administration in insulin-resistant ponies. Am J Vet Res 2010;71:1201–6.

60. Bramford NJ, Potter SJ, Harris PA, et al. Breed differences in insulin sensitivity and insulinemic responses to oral glucose in horses and ponies of moderate body condition score. Domest Anim Endocrinol 2014;47:101–7.

61. Schuver A, Frank N, Chameroy KA, et al. Assessment of insulin and glucose dynamics by using an oral sugar test in horses. J Equine Vet Sci 2014;34:465–70.

62. Borer KE, Bailey SR, Menzies-Gow NJ, et al. Effect of feeding glucose, fructose and inulin on blood glucose and insulin concentrations in normal ponies and those predisposed to laminitis. J Anim Sci 2012;90:3003–11.

63. Bertin FR, Sojka-Kritchevsky JE. Comparison of a 2-step insulin-response test to conventional insulin-sensitivity testing in horses. Domest Anim Endocrinol 2013;44:19–25.

64. Eiler H, Frank N, Andrews FM, et al. Physiologic assessment of blood glucose homeostasis via combined intravenous glucose and insulin testing in horses. Am J Vet Res 2005;66:1598–604.

Exercise-induced Pulmonary Hemorrhage

Is It Important and Can It Be Prevented?

Eleanor J. Crispe, BVMS, PhD[a],
Guy D. Lester, BVMS, PhD, Dipl ACVIM (LAIM)[b],*

KEYWORDS

- Exercise-induced pulmonary hemorrhage • Furosemide • Tracheobronchoscopy

KEY POINTS

- Exercise-induced pulmonary hemorrhage (EIPH) is a common condition of horses undergoing strenuous exercise.
- Racing in cold weather increases the risk of EIPH.
- In competitive Thoroughbred racing, EIPH may negatively affect performance when severe, but this occurs in a small number of competitors.
- Within individual horses, EIPH often is erratic in consistency, although there is evidence that the disease is weakly progressive over a race career.
- Management factors, including avoidance of cold weather racing, increasing the intervals between races, and altering the racing strategy, may reduce the risk of EIPH.

Exercise-induced pulmonary hemorrhage (EIPH) is a highly prevalent disease of racehorses worldwide. Recognized for centuries, there have been solid advances in knowledge and understanding of the disease, but the cause and prevention remain elusive. In the past decade, there have been novel risk factors reported that potentially could be manipulated to reduce the incidence and severity of EIPH. There also have been important advances in understanding of disease progression and the impact of EIPH on race day and career performance. Some of these findings are not necessarily aligned with conventional opinions about the disease and are highlighted as discussion points.

The precise cause of EIPH is yet to be fully elucidated, but a well-accepted theory is that pulmonary capillaries rupture in response to the extremely high intravascular

Disclosure Statement: This article was funded through grants from Racing and Wagering Western Australia and Racing Australia.
[a] Simon Miller Racing, PO Box 7298, Shenton Park, Western Australia 6008, Australia;
[b] Department of Large Animal Clinical Sciences, College of Veterinary Medicine, University of Florida, Box 100136, Gainesville, FL 32610-0136, USA
* Corresponding author.
E-mail address: lesterg@ufl.edu

pressure and low airway pressure experienced during strenuous exercise. The blood-gas barrier is ultrathin to facilitate the efficient exchange of gases, but this predisposes to breakage.

PREVALENCE OF EXERCISE-INDUCED PULMONARY HEMORRHAGE

EIPH is described most frequently in Thoroughbred and Standardbred racehorses, but it is limited to neither these breeds nor these specific competitive racing activities. EIPH has been identified in almost every equestrian athletic pursuit as well as racing camels and greyhounds and human athletes, such as marathon runners and cyclists.[1–5]

The prevalence of EIPH within a population of horses varies depending on the method used for detection (epistaxis, endoscopy, or bronchoalveolar lavage), the intensity of the exercise performed, and the frequency and timing of the examination. Population-based surveys of EIPH have been performed frequently in the racehorse, most commonly in racing Thoroughbreds. Epistaxis, or blood from the nares, after racing or intense physical exertion, typically represents the most severe form of EIPH. Most worldwide racing jurisdictions record episodes of epistaxis, and these records are readily available in the public domain, permitting large population epidemiologic studies. The prevalence of epistaxis after racing reported from these studies ranges between 0.15% and 0.84% of race starters.[6,7] In contrast, the prevalence of EIPH detected using tracheobronchoscopy within 120 minutes of racing is between 44% and 75%.[8–14] The discrepancy in tracheobronchoscopic prevalence of EIPH among studies can be explained, in part, by study methodology (incomplete vs complete visualization of the trachea), the timing of the examination, and the exercise intensity. Tracheobronchoscopic examination of horses after breezing, which is essentially a training gallop, reports a lower prevalence of EIPH, whereas examinations performed after racing, a more strenuous and competitive form of exercise, report a higher prevalence.[9] The time between racing and examination also affects EIPH prevalence. The rostral movement of blood to the trachea is a time-dependent and volume-dependent process, and examinations conducted too soon after racing can underestimate disease prevalence.[12] The population prevalence of tracheobronchoscopic EIPH increases if horses are examined on multiple occasions.[11,15] A recent study reported that 100% of horses that had been followed over a minimum of 7 observations had some EIPH.[15]

Bronchoalveolar lavage (BAL) is considered by some to be the most sensitive indicator of EIPH, with 90% to 100% of horses having evidence of EIPH on BAL fluid cytology.[16,17] This is reflected by the presence of free red blood cells (RBCs) or hemosiderin-laden macrophages.

THE PITFALLS OF ESTABLISHING A DIAGNOSIS OF EXERCISE-INDUCED PULMONARY HEMORRHAGE

There is no gold standard test for the diagnosis of EIPH, and each diagnostic modality has clear benefits and limitations. The best accepted method for EIPH detection is tracheobronchoscopy conducted 30 minutes to 120 minutes after exercise, preferably after competitive racing (**Fig. 1**). Visual verification of blood in the trachea is considered conclusive evidence of EIPH. Given the subjective nature of this observation, scoring systems have been developed to semiquantitate the volume of blood present. The most widely accepted scoring system for tracheobronchoscopy with good inter-observer reliability was described by Hinchcliff and colleagues.[18] The advantage of this 0 to 4 scoring scale is that numerous studies have used the system, allowing for direct comparisons among different populations of horses.[13,15,19,20] In addition,

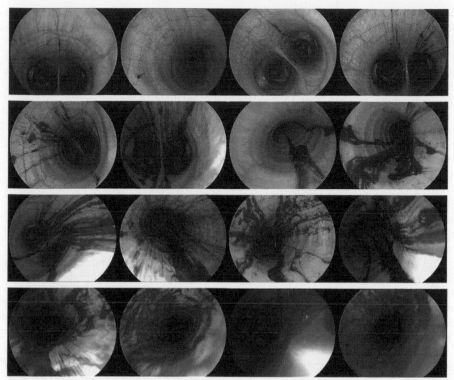

Fig. 1. A collage of endoscopic images demonstrating increasing severity from EIPH grade 0 (*top left*) through to EIPH grade 4 (*bottom right*). Read horizontally from left to right, and down across all 4 rows.

the volume and distribution of pulmonary hemorrhage that underpins these scores are not known. There are no reported limitations of this scoring system. From a user perspective, however, there can be overlap between scores and their descriptions. For example, horses with multiple coalescing streams of blood, covering more than one-third of the trachea but less than 90% of the tracheal surface (grade 3), can have blood pooling at the thoracic inlet, a characteristic limited to grade 4 horses only.

Tracheobronchoscopy is highly specific but has questionable sensitivity.[17] Failure to detect blood in the trachea can be attributed to an inadequate examination of the airways, examination too soon or too late after exercise, an inadequate or inappropriate level of exercise, or a minimal volume of blood in the distal airway that does not reach the trachea.[21] Tracheobronchoscopic EIPH scores can vary markedly from one race start to the next.[15] A high grade of EIPH (grade 3 or 4) diagnosed on 1 occasion does not guarantee high grades at subsequent race starts, and horses should be re-examined to assess the grade prior to drawing conclusions about any negative race day performance. In contrast, horses with lower grades of EIPH are more likely to have consistent EIPH grades at subsequent race starts, but this also is not guaranteed.

Another major limitation of this diagnostic modality is timing. The optimum time to diagnose EIPH with endoscopy has not been established but is likely to vary depending on the grade, with lower grades of EIPH vulnerable to misclassification due to blood present only transiently in the trachea. In 1 study, when examinations were performed from 13 minutes to 175 minutes after racing, those performed during the early part of this window were less likely to detect blood and thus underestimated disease severity.[12] In a similarly designed study, but imposing a minimum time of 30 minutes (median 48 minutes) between racing and examination, time was not associated with EIPH detection or severity.[22] The most severe EIPH grades (grades 3 and 4) are likely less susceptible to timing constraints, reportedly diagnosed evenly across all time categories, ranging from 13 minutes to 220 minutes.[13,14]

To improve the specificity of tracheobronchoscopy, it is recommended to examine horses on at least 3 consecutive occasions after intense exercise or racing,[23] but this does not increase test sensitivity to 100%.[24] The procedure offers the advantage of being quick and minimally invasive, and most horses do not require sedation.

Lower airway cytology has been advocated as a sensitive method for detection of EIPH. Acutely, the detection of free RBCs, or in subacute and chronic cases the detection of hemosiderophages, is the hallmark of EIPH diagnosis using BAL fluid cytology.[25] Hemosiderophages are detected, however, in BAL fluid from almost all racehorses,[16,17,26] and RBCs have been reported in resting horses, possibly induced by the procedure itself.[27] Consequently, the presence of hemosiderophages or free RBCs typically overestimates the number and significance of EIPH positive horses. Although RBC concentration in BAL fluid increases with exercise and pulmonary artery pressure, there remains no clear quantified correlation with EIPH severity.[17,28,29] There also is conflicting evidence of the relationship between pulmonary artery pressure during exercise and the concentration of RBCs present in BAL fluid.[27,28]

To further complicate the value of BAL fluid cytology in the diagnosis of EIPH, the persistence of hemosiderophages within the airway after a discrete episode of EIPH is not known. Hemosiderophages were present at 28 days and absent at 90 days after intrapulmonary blood inoculation,[30] whereas anecdotally it was reported that hemosiderophages can persist in rested horses for up to a year.[31] It also is speculated that horses with continual but mild episodes of EIPH could accumulate numerous hemosiderophages.[32] The percentage of hemosiderophages retrieved does not reliably correlate with the volume of blood inoculated into the lung[30] nor the volume of blood seen endoscopically.[33,34] A hemosiderin score, based on grading of the color of the cytoplasm of hemosiderophages, was proposed to provide a quantitative evaluation for hemosiderophages in BAL fluid.[24,35] These scoring systems were developed approximately 20 years ago but have had minimal uptake in the literature since that time. Other investigators have used the proportion of macrophages that are hemosiderophages in BAL fluid to distinguish clinically significant from nonsignificant EIPH cases,[34,36] although given the potential problems, described previously, this could be erroneous.

It is not uncommon on tracheobronchoscopy to note hemorrhage from a single mainstem bronchus at the level of the carina. The use of BAL fluid cytology assumes that the bleeding associated with EIPH is similar in volume and frequency between the right and left lung. Typically, the BAL tube is passed blindly, lodging in a terminal bronchus in the caudodorsal lung lobe. In a study of French Trotters, using the comparison of cytology from the left and right lungs, the investigators reported that 56% of horses would be misclassified as false negative for EIPH based on unilateral sampling of the lung.[37] EIPH is not a diffuse disease and is subject to misdiagnosis using techniques that sample a singular site. Furthermore, a small experimental study documenting blind BAL tube placement confirmed placement in a terminal segmental bronchus in the caudo-dorsal lung in most horses, but placement in a lateral segmental bronchus also was reported.[38]

ARE THERE RISK FACTORS FOR EXERCISE-INDUCED PULMONARY HEMORRHAGE?

Several studies have determined that racing in cold weather increases the risk of EIPH.[12,22,39] Strenuous exercise in cold conditions is associated with chronic airway inflammation and bronchial hyperactivity in human athletes,[40] and similar responses have been reported in horses.[41,42] The relationship between airway inflammation and EIPH remains speculative. Cold-induced pulmonary hypertension has been reported in other species but has not been investigated in horses.[43]

The application of 1 or more bar shoes was significantly associated with EIPH detection and severity.[22] The basis of this finding is unknown, but it was speculated that horses with bar shoes had subclinical hoof pain, and this could somehow prematurely increase heart rate and cardiovascular pressures during racing.

Although several studies have reported that race distance is a risk factor for epistaxis or EIPH, the findings for both conditions are conflicting. With respect to EIPH, some studies identified increased risk in races 1600 m or longer,[9,44] whereas others report increased risk of EIPH in races less than 1400 m.[12] Some investigators have failed to demonstrate an effect of race distance on EIPH.

There is a cumulative impact of racing on EIPH or exercise-associated epistaxis reflected primarily by lifetime starts rather than age.[9,12,13,15,45] There also seems to be a short-term cumulative association between the number of days in the current racing preparation and EIPH severity.[15] A small study examining a group of Thoroughbreds returning to racing after prosthetic laryngoplasty and ventriculocordectomy to treat recurrent laryngeal neuropathy identified increased risk of postrace epistaxis compared with the general racing population.[46] No studies have identified an association between EIPH and gender, altitude, or racetrack surface. Other factors that have been investigated, such as track firmness and race distance, have mixed results in the literature, with no clear indication one way over another.

NOT ALL TRACHEOBRONCHOSCOPIC EXERCISE-INDUCED PULMONARY HEMORRHAGE IS ASSOCIATED WITH POOR RACE DAY PERFORMANCE

The analysis of performance in racing is complicated, and there is no consensus for a single or collective objective measurement of race day performance. Many studies rely on handicapping to equalize the chances of all competitors permitting easy comparison, but weight allocation alone is not necessarily enough to compensate for a difference in ability.[14,47] Hence, reliance on handicapping to equalize racing can be misinformed. There are numerous factors that could affect the finish position of a horse, including the race class, the weight carried, age, gender, barrier, jockey ability, trainer ability, the race conditions, if the race distance was suitable, and the abilities of the other horses. Other factors, such as the number of races within a racing preparation and lifetime starts, also affect if a horse wins or places in a race.[14] There is evidence that betting markets efficiently incorporate all public and monopolistically held information into the final market odds or starting price and there is a strong positive relationship between the odds and the likelihood of winning.[48,49] Performance relative to rank in the field based on starting price may therefore be the most efficient indicator of performance.

In the past decade, there have been marked advances in understanding about the association between EIPH and race day performance. If the prevalence of EIPH in a population as high as 75% is considered[9] and then the large number of factors that can have an impact race outcome are considered, it is not surprising that early studies using small sample sizes were unable to detect an association between EIPH and race day performance.[9,11,45,50] But as studies recruited larger sample sizes and broadened their definitions of race day performance, a negative association between EIPH and race day performance developed. Although an association exists, it is not applicable to all grades of EIPH.

In Australia, 744 Thoroughbreds were examined using tracheobronchoscopy within 2 hours of racing.[19] Horses with mild or no EIPH (grades 0 and 1) were 4 times more likely to win (P = .006; 95% CI, 1.5–14.3), 1.8 times more likely to place in the first 3 positions (P = .03; 95% CI, 1.05–3.07), and 3 times more likely to be in the 90th percentile for race earnings than horses with moderate (grade 2) or severe (grades 3 and 4) EIPH. Horses with EIPH finished significantly further behind the winner (P = .002) than horses without EIPH. No association was identified between EIPH and career performance indices, which included lifetime starts, number of wins or placings, and earnings.

Another Australian EIPH study reporting 3794 postrace endoscopy examinations from more than 1500 horses concluded that inferior race day performance was largely limited to horses with severe (grade 3 and 4) EIPH only; these categories reflected only 6.3% of all examinations.[15] Horses with the highest grade of EIPH (grade 4) were less likely to finish in the first 3 positions, finished further from the winner, were less likely to collect race earnings and collected less race earnings, were slower over the final stages of the race, and were more likely to be overtaken by other competitors in the home straight than horses without EIPH. Horses with EIPH grade 3 or 4 were significantly faster over the early stages to midstages of the race and significantly more likely to reduce their speed over the final 600 m compared with horses without EIPH. It was suggested that horses that raced with a positive split, where early race speed exceeds late race speed, succumb to breakage of pulmonary capillaries at an earlier stage in the race, resulting in greater hemorrhage and reduced athletic performance. Separation of poor performance due to EIPH from race fatigue, however, is difficult. A study of barrel racing horses reported that animals with the most severe grade of EIPH were faster than horses without EIPH, a finding that also may reflect rapid acceleration increasing the risk of severe hemorrhage.[51] These theories are supported by evidence that horses that rapidly accelerate on a treadmill reach a higher pulmonary artery pressure than do those that gradually increase to the same speed.[52]

Horses with EIPH grade 1 or grade 2 were more likely to improve their position or overtake competitors in the final 400 m of a race compared with horses without EIPH.[14] It is highly improbable that EIPH confers an athletic advantage; rather, a plausible explanation is simply that horse that are ridden competitively to the finish are functioning at their maximal physiologic limit compared with horses that are eased up over the finishing stages of the race because they are not in prize contention or are affected by interference in the home straight. It was reasoned by the investigators that a proportion of horses that do not finish the race competitively do not reach their pulmonary capillary breaking threshold.

EXERCISE-INDUCED PULMONARY HEMORRHAGE SCORE CAN CHANGE FROM ONE OBSERVATION TO THE NEXT

The EIPH literature is littered with anecdotal comments attesting to the capricious nature of tracheobronchoscopic EIPH severity from one observation to the next.[11,53,54] Until recently, no longitudinal study had been performed describing changes in EIPH grade over time. Examination of 2974 observations from more than 747 Thoroughbreds after racing revealed that the EIPH score varied from one observation to the next, particularly as severity increased.[15] Of horses that were previously diagnosed as grade 4 EIPH, 11.1%, 33.3%, 27.8%, 22.2%, and 5.6% were diagnosed with EIPH grades 0 to 4, respectively, at their next start (**Fig. 2**). In contrast, horses previously diagnosed without EIPH (grade 0), the majority (59%) remained EIPH free at their next observation. Factors that were associated with moving between EIPH scores included the number of days since last racing, ambient temperature, and the weight carried. Increasing the number of days between races for horses with an initial observation of moderate (grade 2) or severe EIPH (grade 3 or 4) was more likely to result in transition to a lower EIPH grade at the next start. Horses with previously no or mild EIPH (grade ≤1) were more likely to move to higher grades of EIPH when racing at a lower ambient temperature at their next start. Environmental temperature is one of the most reliable risk factors for EIPH (discussed previously). For horses previously with an EIPH grade less than or equal to 1, reducing the weight carried in the race was associated with a transition to a higher EIPH grade at the next observation. The investigators hypothesized that reducing weight may have increased the race speed, thereby facilitating EIPH.[15] There also are likely to be unmeasured intrahorse and race factors that could account for the variation in EIPH scores from one race start to another.

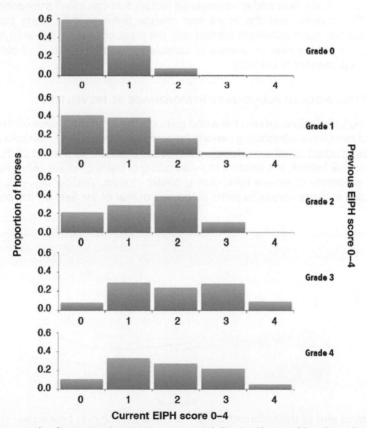

Fig. 2. Bar graphs demonstrating EIPH score variability in Thoroughbred racehorses. The previous EIPH score (0–4) is demonstrated on the right Y axis, corresponding to the current EIPH score (0–4) on the X axis. N = 747; number of observations = 2227. (*From* Crispe EJ, Secombe CJ, Perera DI, Manderson AA, Turlach BA, Lester GD. Exercise-induced pulmonary haemorrhage in thoroughbred racehorses: A longitudinal study. Equine Vet J. 2018; with permission.)

IS EXERCISE-INDUCED PULMONARY HEMORRHAGE A PROGRESSIVE DISEASE?

EIPH has been described as a progressive disease based on histopathologic exami-nation of lung tissue from racehorses. Consequently, the prognosis for future racing typically is considered poor after documentation of a severe episode of EIPH. But a pattern of increasing severity on endoscopic evaluations over time has not been described. Until recently it was unknown if tracheobronchoscopic EIPH severity worsens over time, or if a 1-off episode of EIPH was detrimental to career perfor-mance. It also remains unknown if chronic severe tracheobronchoscopic episodes of EIPH lead to collapse and/or sudden death.

An Australian study retrospectively compared a single observation EIPH score to career performance variables 12 years later.[20] They reported that there was no asso-ciation between any grade of EIPH and career duration, lifetime earnings, or the num-ber of wins or places. The investigators concluded that a 1-off diagnosis of EIPH is an unreliable predictor of overall career performance.

Using a population mean from 2974 horses, tracheobronchoscopic EIPH was shown mildly progressive in severity over the first 30 race starts[15] (**Fig. 3**).

Because there are race and environmental factors that can affect tracheobroncho-scopic EIPH severity, and the score can change between race starts based on extrinsic factors, such as weight carried and the number of days between races, it is unlikely that this marker of disease is suitable to gauge the extent of pathologic change that is present in the lung.

CAN EXERCISE-INDUCED PULMONARY HEMORRHAGE BE PREVENTED?

Many racing jurisdictions around the world do not allow any medications on the day of racing and most have withholding periods for common drugs. These restrictions result in the need to adopt nonpharmacologic methods to attenuate or prevent EIPH. Based on reported risk factors, it is prudent to avoid racing or training horses with a history of repeated moderate to severe EIPH during colder months. Additionally, changing of riding tactics in these horses to settle in the mid or rear of the field off the pace also

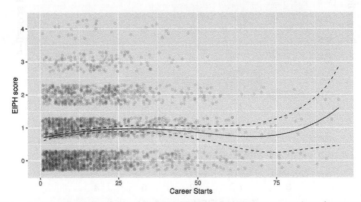

Fig. 3. Jittered plot of tracheobronchoscopic EIPH progression over time (career starts) for 747 Thoroughbred racehorses (2974 observations displayed as individual gray dots jittered around EIPH score to reduce overplotting). The population mean spline is plotted with a solid line and its 95% credible intervals is plotted with a dashed line. (*From* Crispe EJ, Secombe CJ, Perera DI, Manderson AA, Turlach BA, Lester GD. Exercise-induced pulmonary haemorrhage in thoroughbred racehorses: A longitudinal study. Equine Vet J. 2018; with permission.)

may reduce the risk of EIPH. Limiting the number of races in a racing preparation and increasing the days between races also may have a benefit.

Several putative beneficial medications were recently reviewed in a consensus statement on EIPH.[55] The investigators reported that high-quality evidence existed that furosemide decreases the severity and incidence of EIPH. In many jurisdictions, horses predisposed to moderate to severe EIPH are given furosemide during fast work in training. In regions where furosemide is approved for use prerace in confirmed bleeders, horses commonly receive 0.5 mg/kg or 250 mg intravenously, approximately 4 hours before racing.

The consensus statement reported very low-quality evidence that aminocaproic acid, bronchodilators, corticosteroids, nonsteroidal anti-inflammatory drugs, or pentoxifylline reduces EIPH severity. It similarly reported low-quality evidence of a benefit of nasal strips in preventing EIPH.

SUMMARY

EIPH is a common condition of horses undergoing strenuous exercise. In competitive Thoroughbred racing, EIPH may negatively affect performance when severe, but this occurs in a small number of competitors. Within individual horses, EIPH often is erratic in consistency, although there is evidence that the disease is weakly progressive over a race career. There also is evidence that furosemide can reduce both the incidence and severity of EIPH, but, in racing jurisdictions where race day medications are banned, alternative nonpharmacological strategies are prioritized. These include management factors, such as avoidance of cold weather racing and training, increasing the intervals between races, and altering the racing strategy in horses with a history of moderate to severe EIPH.

REFERENCES

1. Akbar SJ, Derksen FJ, Billah AM, et al. Exercise induced pulmonary haemorrhage in racing camels. Vet Rec 1994;135:624–5.
2. Epp T, Szladovits B, Buchannan A, et al. Evidence supporting exercise-induced pulmonary haemorrhage in racing greyhounds. Comp Exer Physiol 2008;5: 21–32.
3. Ghio AJ, Ghio C, Bassett M. Exercise-induced pulmonary hemorrhage after running a marathon. Lung 2006;184:331–3.
4. Hopkins S, Schoene R, Henderson W, et al. Intense exercise impairs the integrity of the pulmonary blood-gas barrier in elite athletes. Am J Respir Crit Care Med 1997;155:1090–4.
5. Hopkins SR, Schoene RB, Henderson WR, et al. Sustained submaximal exercise does not alter the integrity of the lung blood-gas barrier in elite athletes. J Appl Physiol (1985) 1998;84:1185–9.
6. Kim B, Hwang Y, Kwon C, et al. Survey on incidence of exercise induced pulmonary hemorrhage (EIPH) of Thoroughbred racehorses in seoul racecourse. Korean J Vet Clin Med 1998;15:417–26.
7. Takahashi T, Hiraga A, Ohmura H, et al. Frequency of and risk factors for epistaxis associated with exercise-induced pulmonary hemorrhage in horses: 251,609 race starts (1992-1997). J Am Vet Med Assoc 2001;218:1462–4.
8. Pascoe JR, Raphel CF. Pulmonary hemorrhage in exercising horses. Comp Cont Educ Prac Vet 1982;4:S411–7.
9. Raphel C, Soma L. Exercise-induced pulmonary hemorrhage in thoroughbreds after racing and breezing. Am J Vet Res 1982;43:1123–7.

10. Mason D, Collins E, Watkins K. Exercise-induced pulmonary haemorrhage in horses. Equine exercsie physiology. Cambridge (United Kingdom): Granta Editions; 1983. p. 57–63.

11. Birks E, Shuler K, Soma L, et al. Eiph: Postrace endoscopic evaluation of standardbreds and thoroughbreds. Equine Vet J Suppl 2002;(34):375–8.

12. Hinchcliff K, Morley P, Jackson M, et al. Risk factors for exercise-induced pulmonary haemorrhage in thoroughbred racehorses. Equine Vet J 2010;42(Suppl 38): 228–34.

13. Morley PS, Bromberek JL, Saulez MN, et al. Exercise-induced pulmonary haemorrhage impairs racing performance in thoroughbred racehorses. Equine Vet J 2015;47:358–65.

14. Crispe E, Lester G, Secombe C, et al. The association between exercise-induced pulmonary haemorrhage and race-day performance in thoroughbred racehorses. Equine Vet J 2017;49:584–9.

15. Crispe EJ, Secombe CJ, Perera DI, et al. Exercise-induced pulmonary haemorrhage in thoroughbred racehorses: a longitudinal study. Equine Vet J 2019;51: 45–51.

16. McKane S, Canfield P, Rose R. Equine bronchoalveolar lavage cytology: survey of thoroughbred racehorses in training. Aust Vet J 1993;70:401–4.

17. Meyer T, Fedde M, Gaughan E, et al. Quantification of exercise-induced pulmonary haemorrhage with bronchoalveolar lavage. Equine Vet J 1998;30:284–8.

18. Hinchcliff K, Jackson M, Brown J, et al. Tracheobronchoscopic assessment of exercise-induced pulmonary hemorrhage in horses. Am J Vet Res 2005;66: 596–8.

19. Hinchcliff K, Jackson M, Morley P, et al. Association between exercise-induced pulmonary hemorrhage and performance in thoroughbred racehorses. J Am Vet Med Assoc 2005;227:768–74.

20. Sullivan S, Anderson G, Morley P, et al. Prospective study of the association between exercise-induced pulmonary haemorrhage and long-term performance in thoroughbred racehorses. Equine Vet J 2015;47:350–7.

21. Hinchcliff KW. Counting red cells - is it an answer to EIPH ? Equine Vet J 2000;32: 362–3.

22. Crispe E, Lester G, Robertson I, et al. Bar shoes and ambient temperature are risk factors for exercise-induced pulmonary haemorrhage in thoroughbred racehorses. Equine Vet J 2016;48:438–41.

23. Pascoe JR, McCabe AE, Franti CE, et al. Efficacy of furosemide in the treatment of exercise-induced pulmonary hemorrhage in thoroughbred racehorses. Am J Vet Res 1985;46:2000–3.

24. Doucet M, Viel L. Alveolar macrophage graded hemosiderin score from bronchoalveolar lavage in horses with exercise-induced pulmonary hemorrhage and controls. J Vet Intern Med 2002;16:281–6.

25. Hoffman A. Bronchoalveolar lavage: Sampling technique and guidelines for cytologic preparation and interpretation. Vet Clin North Am Equine Pract 2008;24: 423–35.

26. Moore BR, Cox JH. Diagnostic use of bronchoalveolar lavage in horses. Equine Prac 1996;18:7–15.

27. Langsetmo I, Fedde M, Meyer T, et al. Relationship of pulmonary arterial pressure to pulmonary haemorrhage in exercising horses. Equine Vet J 2000;32:379–84.

28. Lester G, Clark C, Rice B, et al. Effect of timing and route of administration of furosemide on pulmonary hemorrhage and pulmonary arterial pressure in exercising thoroughbred racehorses. Am J Vet Res 1999;60:22–8.

29. Manohar M. Right heart pressures and blood-gas tensions in ponies during exercise and laryngeal hemiplegia. Am J Physiol 1986;251:H121–6.

30. Step DL, Freeman KP, Gleed RD, et al. Cytologic and endoscopic findings after intrapulmonary blood inoculation in horses. J Equine Vet Sci 1991;11:340–5.

31. Derksen F, Slocombe R, Gray P, et al. Exercise-induced pulmonary hemorrhage in horses with experimentally induced allergic lung disease. Am J Vet Res 1992; 53:15–21.

32. McKane S, Rose R. Effects of exercise intensity and training on bronchoalveolar lavage cytology. Equine Vet J 1995;27:58–62.

33. Fogarty U, Buckley T. Bronchoalveolar lavage findings in horses with exercise intolerance. Equine Vet J 1991;23:434–7.

34. Richard EA, Fortier GD, Pitel PH, et al. Sub-clinical diseases affecting performance in standardbred trotters: Diagnostic methods and predictive parameters. Vet J 2010;184:282–9.

35. Couetil L, Denicola D. Blood gas, plasma lactate and bronchoalveolar lavage cytology analyses in racehorses with respiratory disease. Equine Vet J 1999; 31:77–82.

36. Newton JR, Wood JL. Evidence of an association between inflammatory airway disease and eiph in young thoroughbreds during training. Equine Vet J Suppl 2002;(34):417–24.

37. Depecker M, Richard EA, Pitel PH, et al. Bronchoalveolar lavage fluid in standardbred racehorses: Influence of unilateral/bilateral profiles and cut-off values on lower airway disease diagnosis. Vet J 2014;199:150–6.

38. McKane S, Rose R. Radiographic determination of the location of a blindly passed bronchoalveolar lavage catheter. Equine Vet Educ 1993;5:329–32.

39. Lapointe J, Vrins A, McCarvill E. A survey of exercise-induced pulmonary haemorrhage in quebec standardbred racehorses. Equine Vet J 1994;26:482–5.

40. Giesbrecht GG, Younes M. Exercise- and cold-induced asthma. Can J Appl Physiol 1995;20:300–14.

41. Davis MS, Royer CM, McKenzie EC, et al. Cold air-induced late-phase bronchoconstriction in horses. Equine Vet J Suppl 2006;(36):535–9.

42. Davis MS, Williams CC, Meinkoth JH, et al. Influx of neutrophils and persistence of cytokine expression in airways of horses after performing exercise while breathing cold air. Am J Vet Res 2007;68:185–9.

43. Greenlees KJ, Tucker A, Robertshaw D, et al. Pulmonary vascular responsiveness in cold-exposed calves. Can J Physiol Pharmacol 1985;63:131–5.

44. Costa M, Thomassian A. Evaluation of race distance, track surface and season of the year on exercise-induced pulmonary haemorrhage in flat racing thoroughbreds in brazil. Equine Vet J Suppl 2006;(36):487–9.

45. Pascoe J, Ferraro G, Cannon J, et al. Exercise-induced pulmonary hemorrhage in racing thoroughbreds: a preliminary study. Am J Vet Res 1981;42:703–7.

46. Mason BJ, Riggs CM, Cogger N. Cohort study examining long-term respiratory health, career duration and racing performance in racehorses that undergo left-sided prosthetic laryngoplasty and ventriculocordectomy surgery for treatment of left-sided laryngeal hemiplegia. Equine Vet J 2013;45:229–34.

47. Verheyen KL, Price JS, Wood JL. Exercise during training is associated with racing performance in thoroughbreds. Vet J 2009;181:43–7.

48. Sung M, Johnson J. Comparing the effectiveness of one- and two-step conditional logit models for predicting outcomes in a speculative market. J Prediction Markets 2007;1:43–59.

49. Vaughan Williams L. Information efficiency in betting markets: a survey. Bull Econ Res 1999;51:1–39.

50. Speirs V, van Veenendaal J, Harrison I, et al. Pulmonary haemorrhage in standardbred horses after racing. Aust Vet J 1982;59:38–40.

51. Leguillette R, Steinmann M, Bond SL, et al. Tracheobronchoscopic assessment of exercise-induced pulmonary hemorrhage and airway inflammation in barrel racing horses. J Vet Intern Med 2016;30:1327–32.

52. Manohar M. Pulmonary vascular pressures of strenuously exercising thoroughbreds after administration of flunixin meglumine and furosemide. Am J Vet Res 1994;55:1308–12.

53. Burrell M. Endoscopic and virological observations on respiratory disease in a group of young thoroughbred horses in training. Equine Vet J 1985;17:99–103.

54. Preston SA, Riggs CM, Singleton MD, et al. Descriptive analysis of longitudinal endoscopy for exercise-induced pulmonary haemorrhage in thoroughbred racehorses training and racing at the hong kong jockey club. Equine Vet J 2015;47:366–71.

55. Hinchcliff K, Couetil L, Knight P, et al. Exercise induced pulmonary hemorrhage in horses. J Vet Intern Med 2015;29:743–58.

What Do We Know About Hepatitis Viruses in Horses?

Joy E. Tomlinson, DVM[a],*, Gerlinde R. Van de Walle, DVM, PhD[a],
Thomas J. Divers, DVM[b]

KEYWORDS

- Theiler disease • Parvovirus • Hepacivirus • Hepatitis • Nonprimate hepacivirus
- Theiler disease–associated virus • Equine pegivirus

KEY POINTS

- Equine parvovirus (EqPV-H) is hepatotropic, appears to cause subclinical hepatitis in infected horses, and could be the cause of Theiler disease in horses.
- Nonprimate hepacivirus (NPHV), a.k.a. equine hepacivirus, is hepatotropic, typically causes mild, subclinical hepatitis and is not associated with Theiler disease.
- EqPV-H and NPHV are common infections in horses and have prolonged duration of viremia; therefore, virus detection does not prove disease causation.
- Equine pegivirus is not hepatotropic and has no known pathogenic effects.
- Theiler disease–associated virus, another pegivirus, is not hepatotropic and has no known pathogenic effects.

INTRODUCTION

Although many causes of equine liver disease are well described (**Box 1**), the etiology of the most common cause of acute hepatitis and liver failure in horses has remained elusive for more than a century. This condition has been called Theiler disease, serum hepatitis, or idiopathic acute hepatic necrosis.

Theiler disease was first described in 1918 as a condition of acute hepatic necrosis that occurred among thousands of horses involved in a vaccine trial against African Horse Sickness (AHS). Sir Arnold Theiler developed a protocol to immunize horses by administering live AHS virus concurrently with serum from recovered horses. In the first trial of 1148 horses, it was noted that 2% developed fatal hepatic necrosis, 4 to 24 weeks after vaccination. However a similar percentage of 4 of 160

Disclosure Statement: Nothing to disclose.
[a] Baker Institute for Animal Health, Cornell University College of Veterinary Medicine, 235 Hungerford Hill Road, Ithaca, NY 14853, USA; [b] Department of Clinical Sciences, Cornell University College of Veterinary Medicine, 930 Campus Road, Box25, Ithaca, NY 14853, USA
* Corresponding author.
E-mail address: jet37@cornell.edu

Box 1
Abbreviated summary of known causes of hepatitis in horses

- Toxic: eg, pyrrolizidine alkaloids, *Panicum* grasses, aflatoxins
- Metabolic: hepatic lipidosis
- Bacterial: ascending cholangiohepatitis, Tyzzer disease in foals (*Clostridium piliforme*)
- Idiopathic: Chronic active hepatitis, (Theiler disease)
- Neoplastic: lymphoma, hepatocellular carcinoma
- New category: Viral: nonprimate hepacivirus (NPHV), equine parvovirus-hepatitis (EqPV-H)

---

local horses that had not received the vaccine protocol also developed fatal hepatic necrosis, and therefore, the condition was initially thought to be a possibly a contagious condition unrelated to the vaccine. The vaccine protocol was then applied to 1411 army horses and 1154 privately owned horses. Between these 2 groups, the hepatitis mortality rate was 4% to 18%, and was clearly recognized to be related to the vaccination protocol at that point. Sir Arnold Theiler reported on the liver condition, which consisted of severe centrilobular to massive hepatic necrosis, and it became known as Theiler disease or serum hepatitis.[1] Subsequently, a similar vaccination approach was undertaken in the western United States to stop the spread of western equine encephalitis, and a similar secondary outbreak of liver disease was observed in the region.[2]

Since those 2 initial large-scale outbreaks of Theiler disease, the condition has been reported in many countries across the globe in association with the administration of a wide variety of equine biologic products. Implicated biologic products include tetanus antitoxin,[3–9] botulinum antitoxin,[10] antiserum against *Streptococcus equi*,[4,11] pregnant mare's serum,[4] equine plasma,[1,2,5,9,12] and most recently, allogeneic stem cells.[9] However, it also has been reported in the absence of any history of equine biologic product administration, and in horses that are in contact with serum hepatitis cases.[1,9,13,14] Collectively, these findings suggested that the condition was both infectious and contagious, and a viral etiology was suspected. Despite intensive efforts by many groups, no viral agent could be cultured from affected animals, and it was not until the recent advances in unbiased deep sequencing that candidate etiologic agents have been discovered. Since 2011, there have been 4 viruses identified in samples from horses with hepatitis, with some discrepancies between the initial findings and follow-up investigations into the pathogenicity of these viruses. The viruses are Theiler disease–associated virus (TDAV), equine pegivirus (EPgV), nonprimate hepacivirus (NPHV), and equine parvovirus-hepatitis (EqPV-H). The objective of this review was to summarize the current knowledge for each of them, what remains to be explored, and the likely clinical implications of infection with each virus. They will be discussed in order of clinical relevance.

THE "HEPATITIS VIRUSES" OF HORSES
Equine Parvovirus-Hepatitis

Equine parvovirus-hepatitis discovery
EqPV-H was first reported in 2018 by Divers and colleagues[15] (**Box 2**). The virus was detected by unbiased next-generation sequencing of liver obtained from a fatal case of Theiler disease.

Box 2
Equine parvovirus-hepatitis
• Virus prevalence: estimated 13% (based on serum polymerase chain reaction [PCR]).
• Seroprevalence: estimated 15%.
• Transmission: iatrogenic through biologic products, otherwise unknown. Viral DNA present in nasal secretions and feces at peak viremia, but actual transmission via these routes remains to be determined.
• Disease association in experimental models: subclinical-to-clinical hepatitis with marked elevations in liver enzymes and function tests, including bile acids.
• Disease association in clinical cases: 27 of 28 prospectively collected cases of Theiler disease were found EqPV-H positive. All cases that had received equine-origin biologics were positive.
• Clinical implications: likely a relevant cause of liver disease ranging from subclinical liver enzyme elevations to fulminant liver failure.

Equine parvovirus-hepatitis viral biology

Parvoviruses are single-stranded DNA viruses enclosed in a protein capsid. The viral genome is small and does not encode for proteins required for viral replication. For this reason, parvoviruses are typically thought to either require helper viruses to provide replication machinery (the Dependoviruses; eg, adeno-associated virus), or to require actively dividing cells such that the virus can use the host replication machinery (eg, canine parvovirus).[16] More recently, parvoviruses have been identified that can activate and use the host DNA damage repair machinery to replicate in nondividing cells (eg, human bocavirus-1).[17,18] The highest viral load of EqPV-H is in the liver, suggesting hepatotropism (unpublished, Tomlinson, 2019). Although the liver is capable of regeneration and cellular division, it is typically a quiescent organ with minimal dividing cells. Therefore, the replication capacity of EqPV-H in nondividing cells is a topic of ongoing investigation.

EqPV-H is one of the few known members of the *Copiparvovirus* genus. Other commonly known pathogenic parvoviruses include canine parvovirus 2 and porcine parvovirus 1, which are both protoparvoviruses, and human B19 virus, an erythroparvovirus. Although the primary tropism of human parvovirus B19 is the erythroid stem cells, it also infects the liver and has been rarely associated with acute hepatic necrosis, although this finding remains controversial.[19–23]

The complete range of transmission modes for EqPV-H is unknown. Iatrogenic transmission of EqPV-H through administration of equine-origin blood products has been demonstrated.[15] However, the virus is also transmitted among horses that have not received such treatments.[14] Although other methods of iatrogenic transmission (such as sharing needles, rectal sleeves, stomach tubes, or dental equipment) are possible, there must also be methods of natural horizontal or vertical transmission. Other blood-borne viruses of horses, such as equine infectious anemia, are mechanically transmitted by biting flies, such as horseflies and stable flies.[24,25] Insect transmission studies of EqPV-H have not been reported to date. No parvovirus is known to undergo biological vectoring in insects, and therefore, tick or mosquito transmission appears unlikely. Preliminary unpublished data (unpublished, Tomlinson, 2019) demonstrate moderate nasal and low-level fecal shedding of EqPV-H around the period of peak viremia; therefore, nasal and/or oral transmission routes are suspected, but have yet to be proven. This remains a high-priority area of investigation.

Equine parvovirus-hepatitis epidemiology

Investigation of the epidemiology of EqPV-H is still in its infancy. Screening of 100 equine serum samples sent to the New York State Animal Health Diagnostic Center for routine regulatory testing revealed a prevalence of 13% DNA detection and 15% antibody detection.[15] All DNA-positive horses were also seropositive. Horses screened for inclusion in experimental infection studies had a higher prevalence of 16 (31%) of 51 DNA detection, whereas young racing thoroughbreds tend to have lower prevalence (unpublished, Tomlinson, Divers, 2019); however, the prevalence can vary widely across premises. Among horses on properties where at least 1 horse has developed Theiler disease, up to ~70% can be infected.[14] Risk factors, such as age, breed, use, housing conditions, and management practices, have yet to be identified.

Experimental infections and herd monitoring show that EqPV-H DNA can be detected in the serum and/or liver for months to years following infection. There is a prolonged period of viremia before seroconversion, which precedes the onset of hepatitis.[15] Although viremia levels decline after the episode of acute hepatitis,[15] the virus often persists at a low levels. Therefore, detecting EqPV-H DNA or antibodies in the serum of a horse with hepatitis might not be sufficient to make an association between EqPV-H and disease. A drop in viremia during the course of hepatitis and resolution might be a better indicator that the virus is associated with the acute episode of hepatitis. However, the full spectrum of disease that can be attributed to this virus and the diagnostic utility of specific tests have yet to be determined.

Equine parvovirus-hepatitis disease association

EqPV-H was first identified in the liver of a case of Theiler disease.[15] A case series consisting of horses with Theiler disease associated with equine biologic product treatment, found that 18 of 18 horses were infected with EqPV-H.[9] Similarly, a case series of horses with Theiler disease without any history of receiving equine biologic products found that 9 of 10 horses were infected with EqPV-H.[14] The other 3 purported hepatitis viruses, NPHV, TDAV, and EPgV, were not consistently found in either group.[9,14] Experimental infection using either EqPV-H polymerase chain reaction (PCR)-positive tetanus antitoxin (n = 2)[15] or equine serum (n = 5, unpublished, Tomlinson, 2018) demonstrates repeatable subclinical-to-clinical hepatitis. Clinical pathology findings have shown significant changes in some horses, including peak bile acids of up to 148 μmol/L; however, no experimentally infected horse has shown fulminant Theiler disease to date. Two major limitations of the current dataset are (1) a lack of case-control data and (2) a lack of purified inoculum for infection studies. In particular, the lack of a pure inoculum has resulted in misinterpretation of previous results from infection studies with TDAV (see the following section), as the used inoculum was later found to be EqPV-H positive also. Therefore, creating a pure, clonal, EqPV-H inoculum should be a priority to definitively prove EqPV-H can cause hepatitis and Theiler disease.

Hepacivirus A, Also Known As Nonprimate Hepacivirus or Equine Hepacivirus

Nonprimate hepacivirus discovery

NPHV was first discovered in respiratory samples from dogs with airway disease in 2011[26]; however, subsequent studies failed to identify the virus in other canine populations (**Box 3**).[27] NPHV is the closest genetic relative of hepatitis C virus (HCV) known to date. HCV is notoriously difficult to study because it does not grow readily in cell culture and known animal homologs have been lacking, until recently. Due to

| Box 3 |
| Nonprimate hepacivirus |

- Virus prevalence: 2% to 7% (based on serum PCR).
- Seroprevalence: ~40%.
- Transmission: iatrogenic through biologic products, vertical, otherwise unknown.
- Disease association in experimental models: subclinical hepatitis with mild elevations in liver enzymes.
- Disease association in clinical cases: 1 report of suspected NPHV–associated hepatitis. Found in only 2 of 28 cases of Theiler disease, and always as a coinfection with EqPV-H.
- Clinical implications: likely a relevant cause of mild liver disease. Capacity to cause clinical hepatitis, liver failure, or chronic diseases, such as cirrhosis, chronic active hepatitis, and neoplasia, is unknown.

its genetic similarity to HCV, species tropism studies for NPHV were undertaken, and horses were identified as the primary host of NPHV in 2012.[27] This engendered excitement that horses could potentially provide a valuable animal model for studying hepacivirus biology. A number of studies have been undertaken to determine the tissue tropism, pathogenicity, and immune responses to NPHV infection in horses.

Nonprimate hepacivirus viral biology

NPHV has also been known as equine hepacivirus[28,29] and is officially classified in the family Flaviviridae, genus Hepacivirus, species Hepacivirus A.[30] Flaviviruses are enveloped, single-stranded positive-sense RNA viruses. They are frequently bloodborne.

NPHV is hepatotropic, as demonstrated by transfection studies,[31] tissue PCR,[28] and in situ hybridization.[32] Although NPHV can be transmitted through iatrogenic blood or serum transfer,[28,33] the natural route of transmission is unknown. Other examples of the Flaviviridae, such as West Nile Virus, undergo complex transmission cycles, including biological vectoring by mosquitoes, whereas other hepaciviruses are not known to be biologically vectored. Vertical transmission has been suggested from 1 of 4 NPHV PCR-positive mares examined, in which NPHV RNA was found in umbilical cord blood and postnatal foal serum.[34] Other routes of transmission or viral shedding have not been explored to date.

Infection in adults typically lasts a few months, but rarely beyond 6 months, with only 4 of 18 reported experimental inoculations resulting in chronic infection (including 7 unpublished, Tomlinson, 2019).[28,31,33] One horse has been identified as persistently infected for more than a decade by testing previously stored serum samples.[31] It appears that adult horses more readily clear NPHV infection compared with foals that become infected when younger than 8 months old,[28,31,33,35] which could reflect a role of adaptive immunity in viral clearance. In humans, persistent infection with HCV is a major risk factor for hepatocellular carcinoma. It remains to be seen if persistent infection with NPHV in horses can result in chronic liver disease or cancer.

As is observed with HCV, there is delayed seroconversion after infection with NPHV. Adult horses typically do not develop anti-NPHV antibodies until 3 to 8 weeks after inoculation.[28,33] In addition, seroconversion can precede viral clearance by weeks.[28,33] Challenge inoculations in 2 previously infected horses, at 5 months after clearing the primary infection, demonstrated a nonsterilizing immunity indicated by a short duration of low-level viremia.[33]

Nonprimate hepacivirus epidemiology

NPHV infection in horses occurs worldwide. The virus has been reported in the United States, Great Britain, China, Japan, and Germany.[32,36–42] The virus is also common: 2% to 18% of adult horses are viremic and 22% to 84% are seroposi-tive.[29,36–38,41,42] Seroprevalence appears to increase with age.[32,38] A history of transportation increased the risk of viremia in horses younger than 8 years old, and decreased the risk in horses older than 8 years, potentially suggesting that transportation increases the chance of NPHV infection earlier in life.[38] Similarly, some of the highest rates of viremia and seroprevalence have been detected in thoroughbred racehorses, although a rigorous test of breed association has not been performed.[32,38,43] In addition, there has been no investigation to date into whether this apparent difference could be attributed to management practices and/or genetic susceptibility. NPHV has been detected in a small number of don-keys, although the clinical relevance was not investigated.[29,36]

Nonprimate hepacivirus disease association

Multiple experimental infections with NPHV have demonstrated only subclinical hep-atitis. Hepatitis typically occurs around the time of seroconversion.[28,31,32] Histopath-ologic changes are subtle and include piecemeal hepatocyte necrosis and subjective mononuclear cell infiltrate.[28,31–33] A consensus sequence molecular clone of the virus was developed and transfected into the liver of a horse. This resulted in NPHV infec-tion and mild liver enzyme elevations: peak glutamate dehydrogenase (GLDH) ~2 times reference interval; peak aspartate aminotransferase 1 time reference interval; sorbitol dehydrogenase (SDH), γ-glutamyl transferase (GGT), and bilirubin increased from baseline but remained within reference interval.[31] The horse had delayed sero-conversion (11 weeks after transfection), and a prolonged course of viremia (19 weeks).[31] This experiment demonstrated both hepatotropism and pathogenicity of the virus. During experimental infection studies, liver enzymes usually increase above baseline without rising above the upper limit of the reference interval, making both detection of damage and interpretation of clinical relevance difficult. Horses demonstrating hepatitis where liver enzymes do rise above the reference range typi-cally demonstrate mild elevations and no clinical signs.[28,31] A longitudinal investiga-tion of naturally occurring infections in Germany identified 2 horses with GGT up to threefold above and GLDH up to fourfold above the upper limit of the reference inter-val; however, horses were not screened for concurrent EqPV-H infection.[32]

One study investigated NPHV infection in a group of horses inoculated with plasma from horses that died of Theiler disease.[28] The horses that died were NPHV positive; however, EqPV-H had not been discovered at that time, and coinfection with EqPV-H was not ruled out. The adult recipient horses developed moderate hepatitis, with peak GGT and SDH 1.5-fold to 5.0-fold above the upper limit of the reference range, but without any clinical signs.[28]

There is a single case report of a horse with chronic hepatitis that was chronically infected with NPHV in Hungary.[40] This case was reported before the discovery of EqPV-H, and it is unknown if EqPV-H could also have played a role.

In people, acute HCV infection is often subclinical and the major health effects are related to chronic infection. There is a definitive need to determine whether NPHV could be associated with chronic liver conditions in horses, such as cirrhosis, chronic active hepatitis, and/or hepatocellular carcinoma.

Pegivirus D, Also Known As Theiler Disease–Associated Virus

Theiler disease–associated virus discovery

TDAV was first identified in a serum sample from a horse with nonfatal serum hepatitis. The serum was deep sequenced for RNA virus discovery, after DNA digestion (**Box 4**). TDAV was identified in the affected horse, as well as in the botulism antitoxin that had been administered to this animal. It was also identified in other horses that had been administered the same antitoxin, but not in other horses on the property or neighboring properties. Only horses that had received the TDAV-positive antitoxin developed hepatitis and were shown to be positive for the virus. In addition, experimental inoculation with the botulism antitoxin resulted in successful transmission of the virus and hepatitis in 2 of 4 ponies.[10]

Theiler disease–associated virus viral biology

TDAV belongs to the family Flaviviridae, genus *Pegivirus*, and has recently been classified officially as Pegivirus D.[30] Pegiviruses are enveloped, single-stranded, positive-sense RNA viruses. Although pegiviruses have been identified in many species, there are no examples of pathogenic viruses in this genus. There is controversial evidence that infection with pegivirus might modulate or attenuate disease due to other lymphotropic viral infections, such as human immunodeficiency virus (HIV) in people.[44,45]

Pegiviruses typically have lymphoid tissue or bone marrow tropism.[46] TDAV also appears to have primarily bone marrow tropism, although intrasplenic transfection with viral RNA was able to elicit infection (unpublished, Tomlinson, 2018). TDAV could not be detected in liver samples from an experimentally TDAV-infected horse (unpublished, Tomlinson, 2018, n = 1).

Iatrogenic transmission through contaminated equine blood products has been demonstrated.[10] No evidence of horizontal transmission from 16 infected horses to 14 uninfected horses was detected over a 1-year period, suggesting horizontal transmission is inefficient at best.[10]

Theiler disease–associated virus epidemiology

TDAV is apparently a rare virus. Aside from the initial report, it has been identified in only 1 additional herd that the authors are aware of (unpublished, Divers, 2013) and rarely in serum samples submitted for viral testing. It has been found in pooled equine serum for cell culture,[47] but has otherwise not been found in epidemiologic surveys in multiple countries and regions.[34,36,41,47,48] In 2 case series of horses with Theiler disease in the Unites States, none of the horses had detectable TDAV.[9,14]

Box 4
Theiler disease–associated virus

- Virus prevalence: less than 1% (based on serum PCR).

- Seroprevalence: unknown.

- Transmission: iatrogenic through biologic products, otherwise unknown.

- Disease association in experimental models: unknown. Experimental infection in 3 horses was confounded by coinfection with EqPV-H.

- Disease association in clinical cases: Not present in any of 28 cases of Theiler disease. Present in a herd outbreak of hepatitis after botulism antitoxin administration; however, horses were coinfected with EqPV-H.

- Clinical implications: unlikely to be a cause of clinical disease.

Theiler disease–associated virus disease association

Although TDAV was suspected to be the cause of hepatitis in the first description of the virus,[10] subsequent studies have failed to identify TDAV in clinical cases.[9,14,15,40] Intrasplenic transfection with TDAV RNA yielded TDAV infection, but no evidence of hepatitis (unpublished, Tomlinson, 2018).

After the discovery of EqPV-H, retrospective testing of samples from the botulism antitoxin–associated hepatitis outbreak revealed that the TDAV-positive antitoxin, horses with hepatitis, and experimentally inoculated ponies were all positive for EqPV-H.[10,15]

Pegivirus E, Also Known As Equine Pegivirus

Equine pegivirus discovery

EPgV was also discovered through deep sequencing of equine serum samples (**Box 5**). In this case, samples were submitted from a group of horses in Alabama, where signs of hepatitis were found in multiple animals.[49]

Equine pegivirus viral biology

EPgV, like TDAV, belongs to the family Flaviviridae, genus *Pegivirus*, and has recently been classified officially as Pegivirus E.[30] Like other pegiviruses,[46] EPgV appears to have lymphoid tropism. Limited tissue analysis by PCR showed that EPgV could be detected in peripheral blood mononuclear cells but not in the liver, spleen, kidney, lymph node, brain, or lung of a single EPgV-infected horse.[28] EPgV has been rarely detected in liver samples from horses in a case series of Theiler disease, even when present in the serum.[9,14]

Iatrogenic transmission through contaminated equine blood products has been demonstrated.[28] Although horizontal transmission has not been demonstrated, the high prevalence of the virus suggests that naturally occurring modes of transmission must be present.

Infection results in a prolonged duration of viremia, which has been documented for at least 17 months.[48]

Equine pegivirus epidemiology

EPgV is a common equine infection worldwide. Approximately 1% to 32% of horses are viremic and up to 66.5% are reported to be seropositive.[36,41,48,49]

Equine pegivirus disease association

Although the source material that led to the discovery of EPgV came from a farm with a high prevalence of hepatitis, there was no statistical association between hepatitis and pegivirus infection.[49] Additional epidemiologic surveys and case series of Theiler disease also have failed to find evidence of a link between EPgV and liver disease.[9,14,48]

Box 5
Equine pegivirus

- Virus prevalence: 1% to 32% (based on serum PCR).
- Seroprevalence: 66%.
- Transmission: iatrogenic through biologic products, otherwise unknown.
- Disease association in experimental models: unknown.
- Disease association in clinical cases: not associated with hepatitis.
- Clinical implications: unlikely to be a cause of clinical disease.

SUMMARY

Clinical Relevance of the Hepatitis Viruses

The story of the emerging "equine hepatitis viruses" is an excellent example of the need for rigorous study and characterization of novel infectious agents. Next-generation sequencing has allowed researchers to identify new viruses that have not been amenable to detection by cell culture methods. This presents the problem that it can be exceedingly difficult to generate a well-characterized, pure inoculum, free of other infectious or toxic agents. In that case, studies rely on the use of samples from clinically affected horses, which can contain additional as-yet-unidentified pathogenic factors. This has occurred in the initial description of TDAV and likely in some of the NPHV studies.[10,15,28] This also emphasizes the importance of follow-up studies to confirm the hypothesized pathogenic effect through case series, as was used to disprove the hypothesis that TDAV caused Theiler disease,[9,14,15] and/or by using alternative inocula, such as transfection with viral genomes, as was done for NPHV.[31] In this light, and although there is strong associative evidence that EqPV-H could be the cause of Theiler disease, additional studies are warranted to further prove the association.

Despite all 4 viruses being described in the context of liver disease, only 2 have turned out to demonstrate repeatable liver pathogenicity. Both NPHV and EqPV-H experimental infections generate consistent evidence of mild-to-moderate hepatitis, although it has to be noted that only small numbers of horses have been infected to date. Consequently, the full range of disease attributable to each virus is yet to be explored. Theiler disease is a rare consequence of equine biologic product administration; therefore, we suspect that individual variation in the immune response may be required to instigate fulminant disease. The risk factors associated with acute liver failure are unknown, just as the consequences of chronic infection are unknown.

Once the pathogenic potential of NPHV and EqPV-H are fully delineated, clinicians will likely still face obstacles in establishing effective diagnostic tests for "viral hepatitis." Because both viruses tend toward prolonged periods of viremia, and horses can remain viremic after seroconversion, a single positive serum PCR and/or serology might not be the most appropriate test to determine whether the episode of hepatitis is related to that particular viral infection. A similar diagnostic problem is, therefore, predicted as what faces us in the context of equine protozoal myeloencephalitis and Lyme disease. Additional tests are likely needed and might include immunoglobulin M serology or serial sampling to document decline in viremia. All this is an area for future research.

To the best of our current understanding, EPgV and TDAV are not hepatotropic and of no direct clinical significance, particularly in the area of liver disease. This is similar to what we know about pegiviruses that infect other species. Additional studies with these viruses should be performed to determine if pegiviruses may interact with the immune system in either a beneficial or detrimental manner, similar to what has been suggested to occur during coinfections with human pegivirus and HIV.[44,45]

Are These Emerging or Expanding Viruses?

Due to the recent discovery of these viruses, their historical prevalence and genetic evolution have only been minimally explored to date. Retrospective review of some herd samples have identified the presence of NPHV as long as 12 years ago[31]; however, older samples have not been screened to the authors' knowledge. Likewise, retrospective testing of serum samples from possible Theiler disease cases have identified EqPV-H in samples from as far back as 1981 (unpublished, Tennant, 2013); so, it is tempting to speculate that these viruses have been circulating in equine populations for decades, at a minimum, and are not truly emerging threats. NPHV appears to be well established in horses across all countries in which NPHV prevalence has been evaluated, and therefore, a significant spread or expansion of the virus seems unlikely. In contrast, the worldwide prevalence of EqPV-H is much less known, due to more recent discovery of this pathogen. It is notable that most Theiler disease reports arise from the United States. If EqPV-H is indeed the cause of Theiler disease, this could indicate a limited geographic distribution of the virus, and a potential that its range could expand through horse movements, shipment of virus-contaminated biologics, or changes in vector ranges, depending on its mechanism of transmission. All this should be investigated in future studies.

Future Directions

Many of the most pressing topics for future studies on these viruses have been summarized throughout this review; however, we would like to propose a few priorities:

- It is essential to confirm the pathogenicity of EqPV-H through additional rigorous study and preferably through experimental infections with purified viral inoculum.
- We need to explore the range of liver diseases than can be caused by NPHV and EqPV-H, and the risk factors that precipitate liver failure versus subclinical disease.
- It will be important to delineate modes of transmission to establish control measures for each virus.
- It would be beneficial to provide more definitive evidence that EPgV and TDAV are not equine pathogens.

REFERENCES

1. Theiler A. Acute liver-atrophy and parenchymatous hepatitis in horses. Union of South Africa Department of Agriculture 5th and 6th reports of the Director of Veterinary Research 1918.
2. Marsh H. Losses of undetermined cause following an outbreak of equine encephalomyelitis. JAVMA 1937;91:88–93.
3. Hjerpe C. Serum hepatitis in the horse. J Am Vet Med Assoc 1964;144:734–40.
4. Rose J, Immenschuh R, Rose E. Serum hepatitis in the horse. Proceedings of the Twentieth Annual Convention of the American Association of Equine Practitioners. Las Vegas (NV): Proc Annu Con Am Assoc Equine Pract; 1974. p. 175–85.
5. Thomsett LR. Acute hepatic failure in the horse. Equine Vet J 1971;3(15):15–9.
6. Step D, Blue J, Dill S. Penicillin-induced hemolytic anemia and acute hepatic failure following treatment of tetanus in a horse. Cornell Vet 1991;81(1):13–8.
7. Messer NT, Johnson PJ. Serum hepatitis in two brood mares. JAVMA 1994; 204(11):1790–2.
8. Guglick MA, MacAllister CG, Ely RW, et al. Hepatic disease associated with administration of tetanus antitoxin in eight horses. JAVMA 1995;206(11):1737–40.
9. Tomlinson J, Kapoor A, Kumar A, et al. Viral testing of 18 consecutive cases of equine serum hepatitis – a prospective study (2014-2018). J Vet Intern Med 2019;33(1):251–7.
10. Chandriani S, Skewes-Cox P, Zhong W, et al. Identification of a previously undescribed divergent virus from the Flaviviridae family in an outbreak of equine serum hepatitis. Proc Natl Acad Sci U S A 2013;110(15):E1407–15.
11. Panciera RJ. Serum hepatitis in the horse. J Am Vet Med Assoc 1969;155(2): 408–10.

12. Aleman M, Nieto JE, Carr EA, et al. Serum hepatitis associated with commercial plasma transfusion in horses. J Vet Intern Med 2005;19:120–2.
13. Tennant BC. Acute hepatitis in horses: problems differentiating toxic and infectious causes in adults. In: Proceedings of the Annual Convention of the American association of equine Practitioners. St Louis (MO): December 1978. p. 465–71.
14. Tomlinson J, Tennant B, Struzyna A, et al. Viral testing of 10 cases of Theiler's disease and 37 in-contact horses in the abscence of equine biologic product administration: A prospective study (2014-2018). J Vet Intern Med 2019;33(1):258–65.
15. Divers TJ, Tennant BC, Kumar A, et al. A new parvovirus associated with serum hepatitis in horses following inoculation of a common equine biological. Emerg Infect Dis 2018;24(2):303–10.
16. Berns KI. Parvovirus replication. Microbiol Rev 1990;54(3):316–29.
17. Deng X, Yan Z, Cheng F, et al. Replication of an autonomous human parvovirus in non-dividing human airway epithelium is facilitated through the DNA damage and repair pathways. PLoS Pathog 2016;12(1):1–25.
18. Deng X, Xu P, Zou W, et al. DNA damage signaling is required for replication of human bocavirus 1 DNA in Dividing HEK293 Cells. J Virol 2017;91(1) [pii: e01831-16].
19. Mogensen TH, Jensen JMB, Hamilton-Dutoit S, et al. Chronic hepatitis caused by persistent parvovirus B19 infection. BMC Infect Dis 2010;10:246.
20. Wong S, Young NS, Brown KE. Prevalence of parvovirus B19 in liver tissue: no association with fulminant hepatitis or hepatitis-associated aplastic anemia. J Infect Dis 2003;187(10):1581–6.
21. Sun L, Zhang JC, Jia ZS. Association of parvovirus B19 infection with acute icteric hepatitis in adults. Scand J Infect Dis 2011;43(6–7):547–9.
22. Bihari C, Rastogi a, Saxena P, et al. Parvovirus B19 associated hepatitis. Hepat Res Treat 2013;2013:472027.
23. Hatakka A, Klein J, He R, et al. Acute hepatitis as a manifestation of parvovirus B19 infection. J Clin Microbiol 2011;49(9):3422–4.
24. Sponseller B. Equine infectious anemia. In: Smith BP, editor. Large animal internal medicine - e-book. 5th edition. London: Mosby; 2014. p. 1060–1.
25. Hawkins JA, Adams WV, Cook L, et al. Role of horse fly (*Tabanus fuscicostatus* Hine) and stable fly (*Stomoxys calcitrans* L.) in transmission of equine infectious anemia to ponies in Louisiana. Am J Vet Res 1973;34(12):1583–6.
26. Kapoor A, Simmonds P, Gerold G, et al. Characterization of a canine homolog of hepatitis C virus. Proc Natl Acad Sci U S A 2011;108(28):11608–13.
27. Burbelo PD, Dubovi EJ, Simmonds P, et al. Serology-enabled discovery of genetically diverse hepaciviruses in a new host. J Virol 2012;86(11):6171–8.
28. Ramsay JD, Evanoff R, Wilkinson TE, et al. Experimental transmission of equine hepacivirus in horses as a model for hepatitis C virus. Hepatology 2015;61(5): 1533–46.
29. Walter S, Rasche A, Moreira-Soto A, et al. Differential infection patterns and recent evolutionary origins of equine hepaciviruses in donkeys. J Virol 2016. https://doi.org/10.1128/JVI.01711-16.
30. Smith DB, Becher P, Bukh J, et al. Proposed update to the taxonomy of the genera *Hepacivirus* and *Pegivirus* within the Flaviviridae family. J Gen Virol 2016;97(11):2894–907.
31. Scheel TKH, Kapoor A, Nishiuchi E, et al. Characterization of nonprimate hepacivirus and construction of a functional molecular clone. Proc Natl Acad Sci U S A 2015;112(7):2192–7.

32. Pfaender S, Cavalleri JMV, Walter S, et al. Clinical course of infection and viral tissue tropism of hepatitis C virus-like nonprimate hepaciviruses in horses. Hepatology 2015;61(2):447–59.
33. Pfaender S, Walter S, Grabski E, et al. Immune protection against reinfection with nonprimate hepacivirus. Proc Natl Acad Sci 2017. https://doi.org/10.1073/pnas.1619380114.
34. Gather T, Walter S, Todt D, et al. Vertical transmission of hepatitis C virus-like nonprimate hepacivirus in horses. J Gen Virol 2016;97(10):2540–51.
35. Gather T, Walter S, Pfaender S, et al. Acute and chronic infections with nonprimate hepacivirus in young horses. Vet Res 2016;47(1):97.
36. Lyons S, Kapoor A, Schneider BS, et al. Viraemic frequencies and seroprevalence of non-primate hepacivirus and equine pegiviruses in horses and other mammalian species. J Gen Virol 2014;95(PART 8):1701–11.
37. Matsuu A, Hobo S, Ando K, et al. Genetic and serological surveillance for nonprimate hepacivirus in horses in Japan. Vet Microbiol 2015;179(3–4):219–27.
38. Reichert C, Campe A, Walter S, et al. Frequent occurrence of nonprimate hepacivirus infections in thoroughbred breeding horses – a cross-sectional study for the occurrence of infections and potential risk factors. Vet Microbiol 2017;203:315–22.
39. Scheel TKH, Simmonds P, Kapoor A. Surveying the global virome: identification and characterization of HCV-related animal hepaciviruses. Antiviral Res 2015;115:83–93.
40. Reuter G, Maza N, Pankovics P, et al. Non-primate hepacivirus infection with apparent hepatitis in a horse—short communication. Acta Vet Hung 2014;62(3):422–7.
41. Lu G, Sun L, Xu T, et al. First description of hepacivirus and pegivirus infection in domestic horses in China: a study in Guangdong Province, Heilongjiang Province and Hong Kong District. PLoS One 2016;11(5):e0155662.
42. Tanaka T, Kasai H, Yamashita A, et al. Hallmarks of hepatitis C virus in equine hepacivirus. J Virol 2014;88(22):13352–66.
43. Badenhorst M, Tegtmeyer B, Todt D, et al. First detection and frequent occurrence of equine hepacivirus in horses on the African continent. Seattle (WA): American College of Veterinary Internal Medicine Forum; 2018 [abstract: E27].
44. N'Guessan KF, Anderson M, Phinius B, et al. The impact of human pegivirus on CD4 cell count in HIV-positive persons in Botswana. Open Forum Infect Dis 2017;4(4):1–6.
45. Bailey AL, Buechler CR, Matson DR, et al. Pegivirus avoids immune recognition but does not attenuate acute-phase disease in a macaque model of HIV infection. PLoS Pathog 2017. https://doi.org/10.1371/journal.ppat.1006692.
46. Bailey AL, Lauck M, Mohns M, et al. Durable sequence stability and bone marrow tropism in a macaque model of human pegivirus infection. Sci Transl Med 2015;7(305):305ra144.
47. Postel A, Cavalleri JMV, Pfaender S, et al. Frequent presence of hepaci and pegiviruses in commercial equine serum pools. Vet Microbiol 2016;182:8–14.
48. Tang W, Zhu N, Wang H, et al. Identification and genetic characterization of equine pegivirus in China. J Gen Virol 2018;1–9. https://doi.org/10.1099/jgv.0.001063.
49. Kapoor A, Simmonds P, Cullen JM, et al. Identification of a pegivirus (GB virus-like virus) that infects horses. J Virol 2013;87(12):7185–90.

Equine Neonatal Encephalopathy
Facts, Evidence, and Opinions

Ramiro E. Toribio, DVM, MS, PhD, DACVIM

KEYWORDS

- Foal • Hypoxia • Maladjustment syndrome • Astrocyte • Progestogens
- Neurosteroids • Neuroactive steroids • Excitotoxicity • Dummy foals

KEY POINTS

- *Neonatal encephalopathy* (NE) is a broad term used for foals (and infants) that develop noninfectious neurologic signs in the immediate postpartum period.
- Controversies about equine NE and neonatal malajustment syndrome (NMS) relate to the lack of pathophysiologic information and target-specific therapies, with most mechanistic explanations extrapolated from other species.
- Based on clinical history, clinical signs, postmortem findings, and recent association of NE with neuroactive steroids, it is likely that NE represents different syndromes with shared clinical features.
- Ischemia/hypoxia and endocrine/paracrine imbalances probably are the main contributors to NE.
- Foals with NE can have abnormalities in other organs that may go unnoticed.

INTRODUCTION

Neonatal encephalopathy (NE) and *neonatal maladjustment syndrome* (NMS) are terms used by equine clinicians for newborn foals that develop a variety of noninfectious neurologic signs in the immediate postpartum period. Since the syndrome was first described by Reynolds in 1930,[1] there have been numerous reports and reviews on this disorder.[1–19] What continues to be lacking is foal-specific mechanistic information because most pathophysiologic explanations have been extrapolated from other species, with few clinical and postmortem studies from affected foals.[12,16,20–24] Dr Peter Rossdale should be recognized as the pioneer in the clinical description, initial investigations, assessment, and management of these foals.[10–14,16] He introduced the concept of NMS[12,14,16] and subsequently proposed a classification of disorders of newborn foals into 4 groups, of which group 2 included disturbances of behavior of

Department of Veterinary Clinical Sciences, College of Veterinary Medicine, The Ohio State University, 601 Vernon Tharp Street, Columbus, OH 43210, USA
E-mail address: toribio.1@osu.edu

Vet Clin Equine 35 (2019) 363–378
https://doi.org/10.1016/j.cveq.2019.03.004
0749-0739/19/© 2019 Elsevier Inc. All rights reserved.

noninfectious nature.[14] Based on gestation and foaling history as well as when clinical signs develop, these foals have also been classified into category 1 (uneventful pregnancy and foaling, normal postfoaling behavior with clinical signs developing 6–24 hours postbirth, and good prognosis) and category 2 (eventful gestation or delivery, placental disease, abnormal behavior at birth, sepsis is common, and poor prognosis).[17,19] Rossdale suggested that NMS was a condition of disturbed adaptation of the nervous and cardiopulmonary systems around foaling.[14] That observation remains relevant today, based on current understanding of endocrine and metabolic imbalances and neonatal brain function.

WHAT CONCEPTS CAN BE UNIFIED ABOUT NEONATAL ENCEPHALOPATHY?

For decades there has been a tendency to group foals with neurologic signs in the immediate postpartum period under a single umbrella, ignoring a range of pathophysiologic processes that could alter brain cell function in the equine neonate. Most of what is assumed to occur in foals with NE has been extrapolated from animal models or people with various acute brain disorders (stroke, trauma, ischemia, hypoxia, and inflammation). In recent years, however, attention has been placed on endocrine and paracrine factors that affect neuronal and glial cell activity in human infants[25,26] but also in newborn foals.[20,21,27] As discussed previously, equine NE can be classified into groups and categories using clinical information; however, trying to unify its pathogenesis is challenging due to the lack of foal-specific mechanistic information on potentially different syndromes with shared clinical features. The goal of this article is to provide a perspective on mechanisms behind the pathogenesis of equine NE, based on information generated from foals but mainly from other species. It is evident from the information presented that the pathophysiology of this condition is far from understood in equine neonates.

The first controversy regarding this condition is the terminology. Terms used in equine practice reflect either clinical signs or presumed pathophysiologic processes. These include NMS, NE, hypoxic ischemic encephalopathy (HIE), hypoxic ischemic syndrome, perinatal asphyxia syndrome (PAS), neonatal maladaptation syndrome, barkers, wanderers, convulsives, and dummies.[1–20,28] NMS, NE, and dummy foal syndrome are considered acceptable terms because they are based on clinical signs and do not assume specific pathophysiologic processes. HIE and PAS may be valid when perinatal ischemia or hypoxia is recognized but may not apply to foals born uneventfully or that develop signs hours to days later. This is supported by the lack of postmortem cerebral lesions consistent with ischemia in several these foals. A similar argument regarding terminology has been ongoing in human medicine.[29,30] In human newborns, HIE is responsible for some but not most cases of NE.[29] Therefore, due to this lack of pathophysiologic understanding, NE has emerged as the preferred term because it does not imply a specific underlying etiology or pathophysiology.[29,30] Moreover, the term HIE, has been proposed to be restricted to animal models where hypoxia or ischemia are well documented.[29] The following points favor using equine NE over other terms: (1) often it is not known when hypoxia or ischemia is the cause of NE; (2) etiologic names may not be necessary when descriptive terms are sufficient to identify the condition referred to; (3) by using etiologic or pathophysiologic names, bias or assumptions are created that are not substantiated; (4) therapies may be implemented based on a pathophysiologic name that may not be appropriate; and (5) this potentially could discourage research based on false notions.[30] Of interest, the use of the NE over the HIE term has been challenged in pediatric medicine, mainly based on information generated from MRI studies, showing similar lesion topography between affected infants and animal models of brain hypoxia.[31]

A second controversy regarding NE in equine practice is that an understanding of its pathophysiology that is not the case often is adopted. Ischemia, hypoxia, reperfusion injury, free radicals, inflammation, hemorrhage, edema, thrombosis, metabolic and electrolyte disturbances, and, more recently, steroid imbalances have been proposed as the key mechanisms in the pathogenesis of NE.[4–24] For foals that suffer ischemia/hypoxia, it can be accepted that the pathogenesis is a consequence of cerebral hypoxia, energy deprivation, hemorrhage, edema, reperfusion injury, neuronal and glial cell dysfunction (cytotoxicity and excitotoxicity), and cell death. The challenge is foals born normally that hours to days later develop neurologic signs. In these animals, it is possible that delayed effects from hypoxia are involved, but possibly metabolic and endocrine imbalances are central to disease development and progression. Ischemia to the brain is easier to recognize than ischemia to other organs with high oxygen demands (eg, kidneys, gastrointestinal tract, liver, and heart). Thus, abnormalities in these organs can be overlooked, or animals may have dysfunction in these organs with or without neurologic signs.

Another controversy regarding NE is whether current therapeutic approaches are effective. Due to limited mechanistic information, establishing effective therapies has major limitations. Treatment of NE is mainly supportive. This opens the question as to whether different therapeutic approaches should be considered (discussed later).

COMPARATIVE PATHOPHYSIOLOGY

In general terms, the mechanisms of equine NE can be dived into (1) those that are consequence of adverse peripartum events leading to ischemia/hypoxia in the prepartum period (eg, maternal or placental disease), at partum (eg, dystocia and caesarian section), or in the postpartum period (eg, umbilical bleeding/compression/clamping, heart disease, and isoerythrolysis); (2) those in which there is evidence or a history of placental disease (placentitis or placental separation) with variable gestation length; and (3) those in which there is no documented maternal disease, gestation length is normal, and foaling is uneventful. Ultimately, the pathogenesis can be separated into ischemic/hypoxic (oxygen/energy deprivation, reperfusion, hemorrhage, edema, and inflammation) and nonischemic (metabolic and endocrine) events.

In foals in which adverse peripartum events are documented, the pathogenesis of NE likely resembles that of other species (ischemia and hypoxia). As previously mentioned, in addition to the central nervous system (CNS), organs with high oxygen demands and metabolic activity (gastrointestinal tract, renal, liver, and heart) may be affected. In foals in which pregnancy and parturition were uneventful or in which there was no evidence of acute cerebral ischemia, it is probable that mechanisms unrelated to oxygen and energy delivery are involved. In these foals, metabolic, endocrine, or neurotransmitter imbalances may be implicated. Within endocrine imbalances, pathways to consider include (1) disequilibrium in systemic and cerebral neuroactive steroids and (2) delayed reduction in endogenous progestogens at the end of gestation (leading to an intrauterine-like dormant state).[32] Either theory could be associated with dysfunction of the hypothalamic-pituitary-adrenal axis (HPAA).[21] Alterations in neurotransmitters, opioids, and cannabinoids potentially are important, but information in equine neonates is lacking.

PATHOPHYSIOLOGY OF ISCHEMIA/HYPOXIA

The pathophysiologic principles of CNS ischemia and hypoxia are shared by animals and people. Therefore, it can be assumed that information generated in other species applies to newborn foals with ischemic encephalopathy but may not apply to foals in which the nature of the neurologic signs is unknown or unrelated to ischemia or hypoxia. The unique endocrine profile of the equine pregnancy is another factor that in the context of foal disorders has been ignored but may play a role in NE. Considering that 20% of oxygen and 20% of glucose consumed in the body are used by the brain, it is evident that interrupting their supply can be devastating. A reduction in cerebral blood flow or oxygen delivery results in glucose and oxygen deprivation, ATP depletion, lactate accumulation, sodium (Na^+)/potassium (K^+)-ATPase failure, increased cell membrane permeability, Ca^{2+} and Na^+ influx, neuronal and glial cell biochemical alterations, cell swelling, membrane depolarization, microglial activation, production of inflammatory cytokines, activation of proteases, reperfusion injury, generation of reactive oxygen species (ROS) and nitric oxide (NO), lipid peroxidation, mitochondrial damage, increased production of neurotransmitters (eg, glutamate), brain edema, increased neurosteroid production, brain cell dysfunction, autophagy, and cellular death (necrosis or apoptosis) from cytotoxicity and excitotoxicity (discussed later).[15,33,34] Reperfusion injury and blood redistribution in response to ischemia have been considered important in delayed lesion severity and disease progression.

INFLAMMATION

Hypoxic-ischemic injury in human infants is characterized by microglial activation and infiltration.[33] Compared with adults, the microglia in the developing brain respond rapidly to hypoxia by increasing phagocytic activity, releasing proinflammatory and anti-inflammatory cytokines, proteolytic enzymes, glutamate, NO, and ROS, which, in addition to causing neuronal, glial, and endothelial dysfunction, also disrupt the immature blood-brain barrier (BBB).[33] This facilitates cerebral infiltration by peripheral leukocytes, worsening inflammation and cytotoxicity. In human infants, neuroinflammation impairs glial cells and neurons resulting in disabilities.[33] In newborn foals, similar processes potentially explain the delay between adverse foaling events and the development of clinical signs. Proinflammatory cytokines have been proposed as mediators of the neurologic signs observed in foals with HE.[15] Other than postmortem examination[16] and 1 study on markers of brain injury,[24] however, information to support this theory is scarce. To add more complexity to the picture, inflammatory cytokines promote the production of neurosteroids (discussed later).

PHASES OF BRAIN INJURY AFTER HYPOXIA/ISCHEMIA

Chronologically, after an ischemic-hypoxic event, cerebral injury occurs in 3 phases, from early reversible (phases 1 and 2) to irreversible (phase 3) states.[35] In phase 1 (primary energy failure; 0–6 hours), neurons are deprived from energy and oxygen, shifting to anaerobic metabolism with lactate accumulation, ATP reduction, Na^+, K^+-ATPase failure, Na^+ and Ca^{2+} influx, water accumulation, cell swelling, edema, cytokine secretion, initial reperfusion injury, ROS production, and cell death. In phase 2 (secondary energy failure; 6 hours to days), the mechanisms to maintain low intracellular Ca^{2+} concentrations continue to fail, leading to glutamate release (discussed later), continuation of reperfusion injury, mitochondrial failure, cytokine secretion, cell necrosis, and apoptosis. In this phase, cell apoptosis continues even when cerebral oxygenation has been restored.[35] In people, phase 2 is the target limit for reversible therapeutic neuroprotection.[35,36] Phase 3 (tertiary brain injury; weeks to years) is well recognized in people, but not in animals, and indicates ongoing inflammation, altered cell proliferation, reduced myelination and axonal growth, epigenetic modifications, astrogliosis, delayed cell death, remodeling, and tissue repair.[36] If similar principles apply to foals, most animals should be in phases 1 to 2 to respond to medical therapy.

REPERFUSION INJURY

Reperfusion injury or ischemia-reperfusion injury occurs when oxygenation returns after prolonged ischemia. The restoration of tissue oxygenation leads to oxidative damage, oxidative stress, inflammation, cellular dysfunction, and cell death (necrosis and apoptosis). Inflammation is a major component of reperfusion injury. In the CNS, reperfusion injury is a key process during stroke, brain trauma, and ischemia. In response to ischemia, hypoxanthine is produced by xanthine dehydrogenase/oxidase. Oxygen is converted to superoxide and hydroxyl radicals. Excessive NO from reperfusion reacts with superoxide to produce peroxynitrite, which is highly reactive. Free radicals, NO, and ROS react with cell components (lipids, proteins, and glycosaminoglycans), altering cell function. Endothelial cells produce ROS to cause additional damage. Leukocytes release inflammatory cytokines and ROS in response to tissue injury. Ultimately, these processes lead to apoptosis. Numerous reviews on reperfusion injury are available. In horses, this is well documented with intestinal ischemia but not for brain or renal injury.

CYTOTOXICITY

Cytotoxicity is a broad term (toxic to cells) that refers to cellular damage or cellular death from substances (endogenous and exogenous), imbalances (endocrine/paracrine and electrolytes), energy/oxygen deprivation (hypoglycemia, ischemia, and hypoxia), immune cells (inflammation), or physical/chemical/environmental injuries (trauma, burns, irritants, irradiation, and pressure). Thus, cytotoxicity may be caused by drugs, toxins, neurosteroid imbalances, neurotransmitters (excitotoxicity), energy and oxygen deprivation (ischemia or hypoxia), immune and inflammatory mediators (antibodies, cytokines, and complement), free radicals (lipid peroxidation or reperfusion injury), immune cells (natural killer cells), trauma, caustics/irritants, and burns. Cells undergo necrosis (fast cytotoxicity: ATP depletion, loss of cell membrane integrity, cytoplasm and mitochondria swelling, organelle disintegration, cell lysis, and phagocytosis by macrophages/glial cells, with an inflammatory response) or apoptosis (slow cytotoxicity: membrane blebbing, cellular shrinkage, nuclear condensation, chromatin aggregation, vesicle formation, cell fragmentation, autophagy failure, and phagocytosis by immune cells, without an inflammatory response).

EXCITOTOXICITY

Excitotoxicity denotes neuronal injury and death from excessive exposure to excitatory amino acids. Because glutamate is the main excitatory neurotransmitter in the CNS, excitotoxicity is primarily a consequence of prolonged exposure to glutamate, which results in cation (Na^+, Ca^{2+}) entry into brain cells (neurons, astrocytes, and oligodendrocytes). Glutamate is continuously released from neurons and removed by astrocytes in an equilibrium (γ-aminobutyric acid [GABA]-glutamate-glutamine cycle) that can be disrupted by reduced ATP supply.[37] Glutamate and GABA uptake, glutamine synthesis, energy generation (lactate production via aerobic glycolysis), and water balance are key astrocyte functions.[38-40] During cerebral ischemia or hypoxia, the loss of energy stores and ATP synthesis alters the ionic balance, increasing glutamate release, but reducing its reuptake by astrocytes.

There are 2 types of glutamate receptors: ionotropic glutamate receptors (iGluRs) and metabotropic glutamate receptors (mGluRs). The iGluRs are ligand-gated cation channels permeable to Ca^{2+} and Na^+ and include the N-methyl-D-aspartate (NMDA), the α-amino-3-hydroxy-5-methyl-4-isoxazolepropionic acid (AMPA), and the kainate receptors. All members of the glutamate receptor family are believed to mediate excitotoxicity; however, NMDA receptors are considered the central players. NMDA receptor activation results in Na^+ (rapid cell death) and Ca^{2+} (delayed cell death) influx. Ca^{2+}-permeable AMPA receptors also play a major role in HIE and are being evaluated as potential neuroprotective targets.[41] Increased intracellular Ca^{2+} activates proteases, phospholipases, phosphatases, proteases, lipases, nucleases, and neuronal NO synthase, resulting in neurotoxic cascades (free radical production, lipid peroxidation, mitochondrial dysfunction, cell membrane disruption, cytoskeletal breakdown, calpain activation, and DNA fragmentation) that affect most cell functions. In other words, glutamate-mediated Ca^{2+} influx seems to be a crucial event in excitotoxicity. In addition, activated iGluRs promote Na^+ and water influx, ensuing cell swelling, edema, and shrinking of the extracellular space.[34] Excessive NMDA receptor activation could trigger neurosteroid synthesis to protect against excitotoxicity.[42] These processes worsen with dysfunction of astrocytes, cells essential for regulation of excessive brain water and glutamate metabolism.[40] The NMDA receptor can be blocked by Zn^{2+}, Pb^{2+}, Cu^{2+}, Mg^{2+}, and ketamine.

During acute brain ischemia or trauma, high glutamate levels also can disrupt the BBB and induce vasogenic edema.[37] The concept of glutamate excitotoxicity has led to the development of drugs to block NMDA and AMPA receptors. Such drugs have been promising in controlled animal studies but have failed to improve outcome in human patients with traumatic brain injury and ischemia.[37] Similar therapeutic principles have been applied to encephalopathic foals (eg, magnesium sulfate [$MgSO_4$] and ketamine), but benefits remain to be demonstrated. The disappointing results with glutamate receptor antagonists have raised questions as to the validity of the glutamate excitotoxicity paradigm. This suggests that the excitotoxicity theory can explain early hypoxic events but not advanced processes that occur during brain ischemia (phases 2 and 3). It also indicates that mechanisms not associated with glutamate signaling likely contribute to excitotoxicity. In support of this theory, the Na^+/Ca^{2+} exchanger has been proposed as a potential therapeutic target due to its importance in cellular Ca^{2+} and Na^+ homeostasis. The $Na^+/K^+/2Cl^-$ cotransporter also contributes to brain cell swelling and edema during injury and can be inhibited by loop diuretics.[43]

THE ASTROCYTE AND BRAIN ENERGY

Although most literature on cerebral energy deprivation has focused on the neuron, there is evidence that astrocyte dysfunction is a major contributor to neuronal failure.[40] Neurons and glial cells have distinct glucose metabolic features, which under normal conditions are coupled (neuron-astrocyte metabolic coupling).[43–46] Aerobic glycolysis and lactate production (Warburg effect) are crucial for energy generation in astrocytes, whereas mitochondrial oxidative phosphorylation (tricarboxylic cycle) and the pentose cycle are more important for neurons to produce energy and maintain antioxidant (NADPH) capacity.[45,46] Because most glucose in neurons enters the pentose cycle, neurons use 3-carbon glycolysis products like pyruvate and lactate released by astrocytes (astrocyte-neuron lactate shuttle) to feed the tricarboxylic cycle and oxidative phosphorylation to generate ATP.[43–46] In neurons, most of this energy is used by ionic pumps to maintain electrochemical gradients as well as action and synaptic potentials. This information supports the key role of the astrocyte as the steady source of energy for neurons.

Relevant to brain injury and ischemia, glutamate accumulation stimulates glucose uptake and lactate production by astrocytes.[46] Glutamate is cotransported into astrocytes with Na^+, which stimulates the Na^+,K^+-ATPase, increasing ATP demand. In addition, the glutamate excess is converted to glutamine (GABA-glutamate-glutamine cycle) that requires 1 ATP per glutamate. In a microenvironment with limited oxygen and energy supply, this glutamate excess puts an additional energy burden on astrocytes, which could have negative effects on neuronal function and survival. Because water homeostasis is a key astrocyte function, astrocyte dysfunction is a major contributor to brain edema and neuronal death. In addition, astrocytes can produce neurosteroids in response to energy or oxygen deprivation.[47] This information could have therapeutic implications in the management of foals with NE/HIE.

PROGESTOGENS, NEUROACTIVE STEROIDS, AND NEONATAL BRAIN DISORDERS

Neuroactive steroids (neurosteroids) include steroids de novo synthesized from cholesterol in the nervous system (central and peripheral, by neurons and glial cells) as well as metabolites of steroid hormones from peripheral tissues (adrenal gland, gonads, and placenta).[21,25,26,48–51] The terms, *neuroactive steroid* and *neurosteroid*, are used interchangeably; however, technically, neuroactive steroids are products of peripheral steroid hormones metabolized by nervous tissue whereas neurosteroids are steroids synthesized de novo in the nervous system.[21,25,26,48–51] They can be classified as pregnane, androstane, and sulfated neurosteroids,[49,50] and their production is dictated by the expression of specific enzymes (eg, 5α-reductase and 3α-hydroxysteroid dehydrogenase).[25,50] Their rapid and nongenomic actions are mediated by cell membrane receptors.[49]

Progestogens and neuroactive steroids are positive allosteric modulators of the GABA type A (GABA$_A$) receptor and to a lesser degree to the glutamate (NMDA, AMPA, and kainate), glycine, serotonin, and sigma 1 (σ1) receptors.[49,51] There also are membrane progesterone receptors (mPRs) in the brain.[52,53] Both neurons and glial cells (astrocytes and oligodendrocytes) have the enzymatic machinery to produce neurosteroids from cholesterol.[25] The GABA$_A$ receptor is considered the main target for neuroactive steroids.[25,49,50] Activation of GABA$_A$ receptors facilitates Cl^- entry, hyperpolarizes the cell membrane, decreases neuronal excitability, and modifies glial cell function.[50] The GABA$_A$ receptor also mediates the actions of several sedative, anticonvulsant, anxiolytic, and anesthetic drugs (benzodiazepines, barbiturates, propofol, etomidate, and ethanol).

Progesterone, 5α-dihydroprogesterone, allopregnanolone, pregnanolone (not pregnenolone), deoxycorticosterone, and tetrahydrodeoxycorticosterone are potent agonists of the GABA$_A$ receptor.[54,55] Pregnenolone and dehydroepiandrosterone (DHEA) have minimal activity over GABA$_A$ receptors; however, their sulfate esters (pregnenolone sulfate and DHEA sulfate) are negative allosteric modulators of GABA$_A$ and glycine but positive modulators of NMDA receptors.[55,56] The sedative and anesthetic properties of progestogens (progesterone, deoxycortisone, and pregnanedione) were described in rodents in the early 1940s,[57] years later in people,[58] and subsequently led to the development of the first commercial steroid anesthetic in 1955.[59,60] Some pregnanes have similar effects in foals.[61] Increased concentrations of neuroactive steroids have been documented in hospitalized foals.[20,21,27]

In people, neurosteroid imbalances have been associated with psychiatric, behavioral, cognitive, and sleep disorders (mood, anxiety, aggression, depression, schizophrenia, premenstrual syndrome, postpartum depression, insomnia, autism, and others).[50] This understanding of pregnane biology has been used to develop the next generation of sedative, anesthetic, anxiolytic, antidepressant, and antiepileptic drugs (eg, alfaxalone/alfaxolone/alfadolone, hydroxydione, isopregnanolone, brexanolone, eltanolone, ganaxolone, minaxolone, and renanolone).[26,48–50] Based on current comparative information on neurosteroid biology, as well as studies showing increased progestogen concentrations in sick foals,[20,21,27] it is reasonable to assume that they may play a role in NE.

NEUROSTEROID FUNCTIONS

Neuroactive steroids modulate $GABA_A$, NMDA, AMPA, glycine, mPR, and $\sigma1$ receptors, promote neurogenesis, synaptogenesis, myelinogenesis, and neuronal plasticity, regulate axon and dendrite growth, alter neuronal excitability, organize neuronal circuits (eg, maternal behavior and fetal brain programming), contribute to glial cell development and function, are neuroprotective, promote energy conservation, modulate the HPAA and the stress response, and are involved in sexual dimorphism.[25,26] Allopregnanolone and pregnanolone (the epimer of allopregnanolone) mediate the sedated state of the fetus.[25,62] Relevant to fetal development, neurosteroids attenuate the fetal response to stress during pregnancy and protect against the adverse effects of glucocorticoid excess on brain programming.[25] Prenatal stress and fetal brain programming are relevant to mental disorders in children and adults.[25,50] Similar events could be pertinent to the equine neonate considering that major adrenocortical endocrine changes (progestogen:glucocorticoid balance) occur in the last week of pregnancy.[32]

STEROIDS AND THE DEVELOPING FETUS

Circulating steroids can readily cross the BBB to be converted by neurons and glial cells into neuroactive steroids.[63] In primates, placental progesterone is the main substrate for steroids produced in the brain whereas in equids other pregnanes and androstenes are likely metabolized. Neuroactive steroids, in particular allopregnanolone, are very high in the fetal brain.[26] Allopregnanolone increases during human pregnancy to promote fetal brain development and programming, to protect from stress and glucocorticoid-induced injury, and to modulate oxytocin release.[26] These steroids suppress brain activity and maintain the fetus in a sleeplike state while neurons and glial cells develop and differentiate.[26] By suppressing excitability, the fetal brain is also protected from hypoxic-ischemic injury.[26] A similar process is likely to occur in equine fetuses because allopregnanolone concentrations are very high in term pregnant mares.[64] During acute fetal stress, for example, allopregnanolone increases to support trophic development (myelinogenesis, synaptogenesis, and apoptosis) whereas in chronic fetal stress (eg, restricted intrauterine growth), neuroactive steroids are inappropriately low (in part due to high glucocorticoids), altering neuronal and glial cell differentiation, brain development, impairing the stress response, which ultimately results in a multitude postnatal complications.[25,26] Excessive glucocorticoid exposure could change the excitatory and inhibitory architecture of the fetal brain.[25] Progestogens also protect brain cells against ischemia, hypoxia, and apoptosis during hypoxic-ischemic encephalopathy, which is relevant to the equine neonate.[65] Cerebral hypoxia stimulates neurosteroid production and hypoxic-induced brain damage is more severe when brain neurosteroid levels are low.[26]

GABAergic neurons project to the paraventricular nucleus to modulate corticotropin-releasing hormone secretion and the HPAA.[25] Excessive prenatal stress could reduce the number of GABA$_A$ receptors, which could indirectly enhance HPAA activity.[25] HPAA activation with increased progestogens is a frequent finding in critically ill and NE foals.[21] Neurosteroid modulation of the HPAA during perinatal stress in part is mediated through opioid signaling.[25,26]

In regard to traumatic brain injury, progesterone and allopregnanolone also have protective and healing actions.[66] These actions are indirect through glial cells (oligodendrocytes and astrocytes).[65] Moreover, progesterone administration to human infants has been proposed as a potential treatment of prenatal hypoxic insults.[26,65] Several studies have shown that progesterone and allopregnanolone can modulate cerebral inflammation, astroglial reactivity, and the expression of aquaporin 4 channels.[67] Early NMDA receptor activation during injury stimulates neurosteroid synthesis to protect against excitotoxicity.[42]

It can be speculated that increased glucocorticoid concentrations, as occurs in critically ill foals,[21] may interfere indirectly with the protective actions of neurosteroids, favoring neurologic disease. It also is possible that these foals have increased progestogen concentrations as a neuroprotective mechanism.

Other factors that potentially are involved in equine NE include oxytocin, endocannabinoids, and endogenous opioids (K. Dembek, DVM, PhD/R. Toribio, DVM, MS, PhD, unpublished observation, 2018).

ENDOCRINOLOGY OF THE EQUINE PLACENTA AND ITS RELEVANCE TO NEONATAL ENCEPHALOPATHY

Fetal, placental, and maternal diseases may contribute to steroid imbalances in the equine neonate. The endocrinology of equine pregnancy is unique compared with other species.[68,69] In the pregnant mare, progesterone and 17α-hydroxyprogesterone concentrations increase and remain elevated until week 25 when they decrease to negligible values.[68,70] As pregnancy advances, other progestogens (pregnenolone, 5α-dihydroprogesterone, and allopregnanolone) rise steadily, reflecting fetal gonad size, adrenocortical function, and placental enzymatic activity.[71] Pregnenolone is the main pregnane in equine fetal circulation whereas 5α-dihydroprogesterone and allopregnanolone are the major ones in uterine circulation, supporting increased placental 5α-reductase activity.[64,68–73] The equine fetal gonads are the main source of pregnenolone throughout gestation, whereas the fetal adrenal glands are the chief contributors to progesterone in fetal circulation.[72] In addition to progestogens, the fetal gonads also produce androgens (DHEA) that are converted to estrogens by the fetoplacental unit.[64,68–72]

Progestogens (pregnenolone) are the main products of the equine fetal adrenal gland; however, 5 days to 7 days before foaling, there is an enzymatic shift from progestogen to glucocorticoid synthesis, reflected as a drop in progestogens with a parallel increase in fetal corticotropin and cortisol concentrations, indicating maturation of the HPAA.[32] Interference with fetoplacental or adrenocortical function could keep progestogen concentrations elevated, delaying the neonate postpartum arousing response, with implications to fetal to neonatal transition and adaptation to extrauterine life. In support of this concept as it relates to placental disease, blockade of 5α-reductase activity in late pregnant mares increases progesterone concentrations.[69,74]

It can be proposed that in the equine fetus, progestogens, in addition to promoting neuronal and glial cell differentiation and plasticity, induce a sleeplike state to reduce energy demands and physical activity. It is documented that allopregnanolone has sedative properties in foals.[61] In addition, increased concentrations of pregnenolone, progesterone, 17α-hydroxyprogesterone, allopregnanolone, androstenedione, and DHEA sulfate have been measured in critically ill, premature, and NMS foals.[20,21,27,75]

Several of these foals also had HPAA dysfunction.[21] The mechanisms that inhibit excessive equine fetal locomotion at the end of pregnancy require precise coordination during labor for proper transition to post-natal consciousness, rapid ambulation, and ability to nurse promptly after birth.[76] It appears that neurosteroids are central to these events. It also can be speculated that the observed signs (depression, recumbency, disorientation, and convulsions) depend on the pregnane, androgen, or sulfated steroid ratio.[75] The association of NE/NMS with high progestogen concentrations suggests that a failure in the transition to consciousness at birth could contribute to its pathogenesis.[20,21,27,75]

RISK FACTORS

Risk factors for equine NE/NMS are maternal, placental, and fetal in nature. Any maternal condition resulting in systemic inflammation or ischemia/hypoxia can impair perfusion to the uteroplacental unit. Placental diseases (placentitis and placental separation) can potentially lead to NE by interfering with nutrient and oxygen supply to the fetus. However, evidence that placental pathologies are strongly associated with NE/NMS is minimal. Microorganisms can be translocated to fetal circulation predisposing to sepsis. Fetal factors include congenital anomalies, twins, prematurity/dysmaturity, sepsis, umbilical cord compression, and dystocia.

CLINICAL SIGNS

Documented clinical signs of NE include disorientation, wandering, lack of affinity for the mare, abnormal udder seeking, lack of suckle reflex, suckling on objects, hyperexcitability, ataxia, tremors, star-gazing, chewing movements, dysphagia, head-pressing, arched neck, blindness, tongue protrusion, recumbency, convulsions, recurrent seizures, expiratory noises (barkers), abnormal respiratory patterns, hemorrhagic retina, hypoventilation, and hypothermia.[1-19] These signs could be accompanied with gastrointestinal (retained meconium, ileus, enteritis, colitis, and diarrhea), cardiac (dysrhythmias), renal (oliguria to anuria), and hepatic (increased liver enzymes) signs.[7,8,15-19] Sepsis secondary to failure of transfer of passive immunity and bacterial translocation is a major and frequent complication.

The prognosis for foals with NE depends on whether they are in category 1 or 2 but also on major complications, such as sepsis. In human infants, the Apgar score is used to assess the severity of brain injury. This score has been modified to evaluate mentation and prognosis for survival in newborn foals.

LABORATORY FINDINGS

Reported laboratory abnormalities in foals with NE include hypoxemia, hypercapnia, acidemia, hyperlactatemia, azotemia, hypoglycemia, hypocalcemia, hypomagnesemia, hypermagnesemia, and low thyroid hormone concentrations.[7,8,10,15,20,21,23,77,78] Most of these abnormalities are secondary to systemic disease (sepsis and hypoperfusion) and organ dysfunction and not a direct manifestation of NE. High total calcium concentration and low alkaline phosphate activity have been linked with survival in foals with NE.[8] The use of inotropes, suggesting tissue hypoperfusion, was associated with mortality.[8] Examination of cerebrospinal fluid is not routine, but it could be normal, xanthochromic, or hemorrhagic.

DIAGNOSIS

Determining the cause of NE can be challenging. A diagnosis is reached from the clinical history, clinical signs but more often by exclusion of infectious and congenital conditions.[8] As discussed previously, many of these foals appear normal at birth but develop neurologic signs hours later. Laboratory abnormalities reflect perinatal diseases more than NE. Blood markers of brain injury, such as ubiquitin C-terminal hydrolase, have been measured for research purposes but have limited clinical value.[24] Imaging, such as MRI and electroencephalography, may have diagnostic and prognostic value in some foals.[4,79]

TREATMENTS, RATIONALE, AND EVIDENCE OF SUCCESS

Drugs used to treat foals with NE/NMS include diazepam, midazolam, phenobarbital, $MgSO_4$, ketamine, naloxone, doxapram, caffeine, thiamine, ascorbic acid, vitamin E, dimethyl sulfoxide, furosemide, mannitol, allopurinol, fenoldopam, pentoxifylline, hetastarch, hypertonic saline solution, and oxygen insufflation. Hyperbaric oxygen therapy has been used in some cases. Support therapy is necessary and dictated by the clinical presentation, laboratory abnormalities, and prevention of complications. Colostrum or plasma administration are indicated because failure of transfer of passive immunity is frequent in these foals. Antimicrobial drugs must be part of the therapeutic protocol due to their high risk for sepsis from in utero infections, intestinal bacterial translocation, and low IgG concentrations.

It is important to note that with supportive care the majority of these foals will recover without residual neurological deficits. Cost of treatment is variable, depending on a multitude of factors, in particular associated complications.

Therapies evaluated in human infants with HIE/NE include hypothermia, erythropoietin, melatonin, xenon, topiramate, azithromycin, allopurinol, $MgSO_4$, Insulin-like growth factor-1, monosialoganglioside, docosahexaenoic acid, and stem cells.[35,36,80,81] Agents investigated in preclinical models of HIE include argon, cannabinoids, osteopontin, edaravone, and interferon-β.[35,36,80,81] Hypothermia is the only intervention shown to reduce death and disabilities in human neonates with HIE, and it is considered the standard of care.[29] Xenon is a general anesthetic with high affinity for NMDA receptors, is not neurotoxic, protects against ischemia, and it is being evaluated in clinical trials of NE with promising results. Ganaxolone is a synthetic by-product of allopregnanolone that seems effective at controlling neonatal seizures. Because Mg^{2+} blocks Ca^{2+} channels and inhibits NMDA receptors, $MgSO_4$ has been evaluated in clinical trials of human adults with acute brain injury as well as in infants with NE/HIE, with variable results.[54] $MgSO_4$ also is used in foals with NE; however, efficacy has not been demonstrated in retrospective or prospective studies. Of interest, 1 study found that foals with PAS had higher total magnesium concentrations than healthy and septic foals.[22] Ketamine is occasionally used under the same principle of blocking NMDA receptors.

A squeeze procedure has been advocated to mimic the fetal neural reflex that occurs in the birth canal during the transition from intrauterine unconsciousness to extrauterine awareness.[82,83] Success with this technique has been variable, although a survey found faster recoveries in NE foals receiving the squeeze procedure for 20 minutes This is a safe method to consider in foals without evidence of perinatal ischemia.[82]

Although there are foals in which some of these therapies may improve outcome, consensus on which is the most effective treatment is lacking. A good example is oxygen insufflation—by the time it is instituted is usually too late to make a difference, except for those foals with cardiorespiratory compromise.

Under the premise that increased allopregnanolone synthesis contributes to NE, 5α-reductase inhibitors (finasteride and dutasteride) have been administered to foals with NE N.M. Slovis, DVM, personal communication, 2018; however, benefits are unclear. As discussed previously, increased allopregnanolone during brain injury is considered neuroprotective and its manipulation could have unintended effects. Allopregnanolone analogs currently are used to control seizures in adults and children.[50,51,66,84] Therefore, a better understanding on neurosteroid biology will lead to better therapeutic interventions for foals with NE.

NECROPSY FINDINGS

Reported gross findings include congestion, hemorrhage, edema, and necrosis in different regions of the brain. Microscopically, there is swelling, edema, necrosis, and malacia as well as neuronal and glial cell necrosis and apoptosis. Many of these lesions are similar to those seen in animals subjected to experimental ischemia. It is important, however, to mention that neuronal and glial necrosis do not necessarily imply ischemia/hypoxia but could be a result of excitotoxicity or inflammation. Several foals with signs of NE have minimal to no lesions to explain their clinical signs. Many of the foals in the study by Palmer and Rossdale[16] had uneventful births, suggesting that other mechanisms triggered many of the postmortem lesions found. Lesions in other organs are variable, depending on duration of clinical signs and complications (eg, sepsis, hypoperfusion).

SUMMARY

Equine NE refers to several noninfectious neurologic conditions of newborn foals. Based on clinical history and findings, NE seems to cover different syndromes. The terms NE and NMS do not assume an understanding of the etiology or pathogenesis leading to the clinical presentation of this condition. Ischemia/hypoxia and endocrine imbalances (progestogens, neurosteroids) probably are major contributors to equine NE; however, mechanistic research is necessary to provide corroboration. There are controversies about its pathophysiology and what are the best specific therapies. There is consensus, however, that treatment should be directed at the clinical signs and complications. Dysfunction in organs with high oxygen demand can go unnoticed.

REFERENCES

1. Reynolds EB. Clinical notes on some conditions met within the mare following parturition and in the newly born foal. Vet Rec 1930;10:277–80.
2. Baird JD. Neonatal maladjustment syndrome in a thoroughbred foal. Aust Vet J 1973;49:530–4.
3. Cosgrove JSM. The veterinary surgeon and the newborn foal. Vet Rec 1955;97:967.
4. Dickey EJ, Long SN, Hunt RW. Hypoxic ischemic encephalopathy–what can we learn from humans? J Vet Intern Med 2011;25:1231–40.
5. Diesch TJ, Mellor DJ. Birth transitions: pathophysiology, the onset of consciousness and possible implications for neonatal maladjustment syndrome in the foal. Equine Vet J 2013;45:656–60.
6. Galvin N, Collins D. Perinatal asphyxia syndrome in the foal: review and a case report. Ir Vet J 2004;57:707–14.
7. Gold JR. Perinatal asphyxia syndrome. Equine Vet Educ 2017;29:158–64.
8. Lyle-Dugas J, Giguere S, Mallicote MF, et al. Factors associated with outcome in 94 hospitalised foals diagnosed with neonatal encephalopathy. Equine Vet J 2017;49:207–10.
9. Mahaffey LW, Rossdale PD. Convulsive and allied syndrome in newborn foals. Vet Rec 1957;69:1277–89.
10. Rossdale PD. Clinical studies on the newborn thoroughbred foal. I. Perinatal behaviour. Br Vet J 1967;123:470–81.

11. Rossdale PD. Abnormal perinatal behaviour in the thoroughbred horse. Br Vet J 1968;124:540–53.
12. Rossdale PD. Clinical studies on 4 newborn throughbred foals suffering from convulsions with special reference to blood gas chemistry and pulmonary ventilation. Res Vet Sci 1969;10:279–91.
13. Rossdale PD. The adaptive processes of the newborn foal. Vet Rec 1970;87:37–8.
14. Rossdale PD. Modern concepts of neonatal disease in foals. Equine Vet J 1972;4: 117–28.
15. Wong D, Wilkins PA, Bain FT, et al. Neonatal encephalopathy in foals. Compend Contin Educ Vet 2011;33:E5.
16. Palmer AC, Rossdale PD. Neuropathology of the convulsive foal syndrome. J Reprod Fertil Suppl 1975;(23):691–4.
17. Clement SF. Convulsive and allied syndromes of the neonatal foal. Vet Clin North Am Equine Pract 1987;3:333–44.
18. MacKay RJ. Neurologic disorders of neonatal foals. Vet Clin North Am Equine Pract 2005;21:387–406, vii.
19. Hess-Dudan F, Rossdale PD. Neonatal maladjustment syndrome and other neurological signs in the newborn foal: part 1. Equine Vet Educ 1996;8:24–32.
20. Aleman M, Pickles KJ, Conley AJ, et al. Abnormal plasma neuroactive progestagen derivatives in ill, neonatal foals presented to the neonatal intensive care unit. Equine Vet J 2013;45:661–5.
21. Dembek KA, Timko KJ, Johnson LM, et al. Steroids, steroid precursors, and neuroactive steroids in critically ill equine neonates. Vet J 2017;225:42–9.
22. Mariella J, Isani G, Andreani G, et al. Total plasma magnesium in healthy and critically ill foals. Theriogenology 2016;85:180–5.
23. Pirrone A, Panzani S, Govoni N, et al. Thyroid hormone concentrations in foals affected by perinatal asphyxia syndrome. Theriogenology 2013;80:624–9.
24. Ringger NC, Giguere S, Morresey PR, et al. Biomarkers of brain injury in foals with hypoxic-ischemic encephalopathy. J Vet Intern Med 2011;25:132–7.
25. Brunton PJ. Programming the brain and behaviour by early-life stress: a focus on neuroactive steroids. J Neuroendocrinol 2015;27:468–80.
26. Hirst JJ, Kelleher MA, Walker DW, et al. Neuroactive steroids in pregnancy: key regulatory and protective roles in the foetal brain. J Steroid Biochem Mol Biol 2014;139:144–53.
27. Rossdale PD, Ousey JC, McGladdery AJ, et al. A retrospective study of increased plasma progestagen concentrations in compromised neonatal foals. Reprod Fertil Dev 1995;7:567–75.
28. Mahaffey LW, Rossdale PD. A convulsive syndrome in newborn foals resembling pulmonary syndrome in the newborn infant. Lancet 1959;1:1223–5.
29. Molloy EJ, Bearer C. Neonatal encephalopathy versus hypoxic-ischemic encephalopathy. Pediatr Res 2018;84(5):574.
30. Dammann O, Ferriero D, Gressens P. Neonatal encephalopathy or hypoxic-ischemic encephalopathy? Appropriate terminology matters. Pediatr Res 2011;70:1–2.
31. Volpe JJ. Neonatal encephalopathy: an inadequate term for hypoxic-ischemic encephalopathy. Ann Neurol 2012;72:156–66.
32. Fowden AL, Forhead AJ, Ousey JC. Endocrine adaptations in the foal over the perinatal period. Equine Vet J Suppl 2012;(41):130–9.
33. Liu F, McCullough LD. Inflammatory responses in hypoxic ischemic encephalopathy. Acta Pharmacol Sin 2013;34:1121–30.
34. Xing C, Arai K, Lo EH, et al. Pathophysiologic cascades in ischemic stroke. Int J Stroke 2012;7:378–85.

35. Greenwood A, Evans J, Smit E. New brain protection strategies for infants with hypoxic-ischaemic encephalopathy. Paediatr Child Health 2018;28:405–11.
36. Nair J, Kumar VHS. Current and emerging therapies in the management of hypoxic ischemic encephalopathy in neonates. Children (Basel) 2018;5 [pii:E99].
37. Andras IE, Deli MA, Veszelka S, et al. The NMDA and AMPA/KA receptors are involved in glutamate-induced alterations of occludin expression and phosphorylation in brain endothelial cells. J Cereb Blood Flow Metab 2007;27:1431–43.
38. Westergaard N, Sonnewald U, Schousboe A. Metabolic trafficking between neurons and astrocytes: the glutamate/glutamine cycle revisited. Dev Neurosci 1995; 17:203–11.
39. Brekke E, Morken TS, Sonnewald U. Glucose metabolism and astrocyte-neuron interactions in the neonatal brain. Neurochem Int 2015;82:33–41.
40. Pasantes-Morales H, Vazquez-Juarez E. Transporters and channels in cytotoxic astrocyte swelling. Neurochem Res 2012;37:2379–87.
41. Tang XJ, Xing F. Calcium-permeable AMPA receptors in neonatal hypoxic-ischemic encephalopathy [review]. Biomed Rep 2013;1:828–32.
42. Guarneri P, Russo D, Cascio C, et al. Induction of neurosteroid synthesis by NMDA receptors in isolated rat retina: a potential early event in excitotoxicity. Eur J Neurosci 1998;10:1752–63.
43. Jayakumar AR, Norenberg MD. The Na-K-Cl Co-transporter in astrocyte swelling. Metab Brain Dis 2010;25:31–8.
44. Belanger M, Allaman I, Magistretti PJ. Brain energy metabolism: focus on astrocyte-neuron metabolic cooperation. Cell Metab 2011;14:724–38.
45. Stobart JL, Anderson CM. Multifunctional role of astrocytes as gatekeepers of neuronal energy supply. Front Cell Neurosci 2013;7:38.
46. Magistretti PJ, Allaman I. A cellular perspective on brain energy metabolism and functional imaging. Neuron 2015;86:883–901.
47. Brunton PJ, Russell JA, Hirst JJ. Allopregnanolone in the brain: protecting pregnancy and birth outcomes. Prog Neurobiol 2014;113:106–36.
48. Melcangi RC, Giatti S, Pesaresi M, et al. Role of neuroactive steroids in the peripheral nervous system. Front Endocrinol (Lausanne) 2011;2:104.
49. Tuem KB, Atey TM. Neuroactive Steroids: Receptor Interactions and Responses. Front Neurol 2017;8:442.
50. Reddy DS, Estes WA. Clinical potential of neurosteroids for CNS disorders. Trends Pharmacol Sci 2016;37:543–61.
51. Longone P, di Michele F, D'Agati E, et al. Neurosteroids as neuromodulators in the treatment of anxiety disorders. Front Endocrinol (Lausanne) 2011;2:55.
52. Thomas P, Pang Y. Membrane progesterone receptors: evidence for neuroprotective, neurosteroid signaling and neuroendocrine functions in neuronal cells. Neuroendocrinology 2012;96:162–71.
53. Dressing GE, Goldberg JE, Charles NJ, et al. Membrane progesterone receptor expression in mammalian tissues: a review of regulation and physiological implications. Steroids 2011;76:11–7.
54. Olsen RW. GABAA receptor: positive and negative allosteric modulators. Neuropharmacology 2018;136:10–22.
55. Wang M. Neurosteroids and GABA-A receptor function. Front Endocrinol (Lausanne) 2011;2:44.
56. Laube B, Maksay G, Schemm R, et al. Modulation of glycine receptor function: a novel approach for therapeutic intervention at inhibitory synapses? Trends Pharmacol Sci 2002;23:519–27.

57. Selye H. Studies concerning the correlation between anesthetic potency, hormonal activity and chemical structure among steroid compounds. Curr Res Anesth Analg 1942;21:41–7.
58. Merryman W, Boiman R, Barnes L, et al. Progesterone anesthesia in human subjects. J Clin Endocrinol Metab 1954;14:1567–9.
59. P'An SY, Gardocki JF, Hutcheon DE, et al. General anesthetic and other pharmacological properties of a soluble steroid, 21-hydroxypregnanedione sodium succianate. J Pharmacol Exp Ther 1955;115:432–41.
60. Laubach GD, P'An SY, Rudel HW. Steroid anesthetic agent. Science 1955;122:78.
61. Madigan JE, Haggettt EF, Pickles KJ, et al. Allopregnanolone infusion induced neurobehavioural alterations in a neonatal foal: is this a clue to the pathogenesis of neonatal maladjustment syndrome? Equine Vet J Suppl 2012;(41):109–12.
62. Lagercrantz H, Changeux JP. The emergence of human consciousness: from fetal to neonatal life. Pediatr Res 2009;65:255–60.
63. Belelli D, Lambert JJ. Neurosteroids: endogenous regulators of the GABA(A) receptor. Nat Rev Neurosci 2005;6:565–75.
64. Ousey JC, Forhead AJ, Rossdale PD, et al. Ontogeny of uteroplacental progestagen production in pregnant mares during the second half of gestation. Biol Reprod 2003;69:540–8.
65. Kawarai Y, Tanaka H, Kobayashi T, et al. Progesterone as a postnatal prophylactic agent for encephalopathy caused by prenatal hypoxic ischemic insult. Endocrinology 2018;159:2264–74.
66. Rey M, Coirini H. Synthetic neurosteroids on brain protection. Neural Regen Res 2015;10:17–21.
67. Biagini G, Marinelli C, Panuccio G, et al. Glia-neuron interactions: neurosteroids and epileptogenesis. In: Noebels JL, Avoli M, Rogawski MA, et al, editors. Jasper's basic mechanisms of the epilepsies. 2012. Bethesda (MD).
68. Conley AJ. Review of the reproductive endocrinology of the pregnant and parturient mare. Theriogenology 2016;86:355–65.
69. Fowden AL, Forhead AJ, Ousey JC. The Endocrinology of equine parturition. Exp Clin Endocrinol Diabetes 2008;116:393–403.
70. Legacki EL, Scholtz EL, Ball BA, et al. The dynamic steroid landscape of equine pregnancy mapped by mass spectrometry. Reproduction 2016;151:421–30.
71. Rossdale PD, McGladdery AJ, Ousey JC, et al. Increase in plasma progestagen concentrations in the mare after foetal injection with CRH, ACTH or betamethasone in late gestation. Equine Vet J 1992;24(5):347–50.
72. Legacki EL, Ball BA, Corbin CJ, et al. Equine fetal adrenal, gonadal and placental steroidogenesis. Reproduction 2017;154:445–54.
73. Scholtz EL, Krishnan S, Ball BA, et al. Pregnancy without progesterone in horses defines a second endogenous biopotent progesterone receptor agonist, 5alpha-dihydroprogesterone. Proc Natl Acad Sci U S A 2014;111:3365–70.
74. Wynn MAA, Ball BA, Legacki E, et al. Inhibition of 5alpha-reductase alters pregnane metabolism in the late pregnant mare. Reproduction 2018;155:251–8.
75. Houghton E, Holtan D, Grainger L, et al. Plasma progestagen concentrations in the normal and dysmature newborn foal. J Reprod Fertil Suppl 1991;44:609–17.
76. Mellor DJ. Galloping colts, fetal feelings, and reassuring regulations: putting animal-welfare science into practice. J Vet Med Educ 2010;37:94–100.
77. Bernard WV, Reimer JM, Cudd T, et al. Historical factors, clinicopathologic findings, clinical features, and outcome of equine neonates presenting with or developing signs of central nervous system disease. Proc Am Assoc Equine Practitiones 1995;41:222–4.

78. Rossdale PD. Clinical view of disturbances in equine foetal maturation. Equine Vet J Suppl 1993;(14):3–7.
79. Wong DM, Jeffery N, Hepworth-Warren KL, et al. Magnetic resonance imaging of presumptive neonatal encephalopathy in a foal. Equine Vet Educ 2017;29: 534–8.
80. Martinello K, Hart AR, Yap S, et al. Management and investigation of neonatal encephalopathy: 2017 update. Arch Dis Child Fetal Neonatal Ed 2017;102: F346–58.
81. Muller AJ, Marks JD. Hypoxic ischemic brain injury: potential therapeutic interventions for the future. Neoreviews 2014;15:e177–86.
82. Aleman M, Weich KM, Madigan JE. Survey of veterinarians using a novel physical compression squeeze procedure in the management of neonatal maladjustment syndrome in foals. Animals (Basel) 2017;7 [pii:E69]. Available at: https://www.ncbi.nlm.nih.gov/pubmed/23176413.
83. Toth, Aleman M, Brosnan RJ, et al. Evaluation of squeeze-induced somnolence in neonatal foals. Am J Vet Res 2012;73(12):1881–9.
84. Yawno T, Miller SL, Bennet L, et al. Ganaxolone: a new treatment for neonatal seizures. Front Cell Neurosci 2017;11:246.

Are There Shared Mechanisms in the Pathophysiology of Different Clinical Forms of Laminitis and What Are the Implications for Prevention and Treatment?

Andrew W. van Eps, BVSc, PhD[a],*, Teresa A. Burns, DVM, PhD[b]

KEYWORDS

- Laminitis • Endocrinopathic • Sepsis • Supporting limb • Lamellae • Adhesion
- Basement membrane

KEY POINTS

- There are both unique and shared elements in the pathophysiology of different forms of laminitis.
- Key pathophysiologic events in each form are insulin dysregulation in endocrinopathic laminitis, ischemia in supporting limb laminitis, and inflammation in sepsis-related laminitis.
- These different events converge to cause lamellar attachment failure through adhesion loss and cell stretch, which may be mediated by common growth factor signaling pathways.
- Tissue damage through mechanical distraction, inflammation, pain, and a proliferative epithelial healing response are features of acute laminitis regardless of the cause.
- Preventive and treatment strategies can be based on knowledge of these unique and common mechanistic events in order to improve clinical outcomes.

Disclosure: The presented work is supported by grants from the Grayson Jockey Club Research Foundation, Digital hypothermia in Laminitis: Timing & Signaling, Laminar Signaling in Supporting Limb Laminitis, Events Affecting Laminar Adhesion in Equine Sepsis, Endocrinopathic Laminitis: Pathophysiology and Treatment, Lamellar Energy Failure in Supporting Limb Laminitis, Weight Bearing; Perfusion and Bioenergetics in Laminitis and Prevention of Supporting Limb Laminitis.

[a] Department of Clinical Studies - New Bolton Center, School of Veterinary Medicine, University of Pennsylvania, 382 West Street Road, Kennett Square, PA 19348, USA; [b] Department of Veterinary Clinical Studies, College of Veterinary Medicine, The Ohio State University, 601 Vernon Tharp Street, Columbus, OH 43210, USA
* Corresponding author.
E-mail address: vaneps@vet.upenn.edu

Vet Clin Equine 35 (2019) 379–398
https://doi.org/10.1016/j.cveq.2019.04.001
0749-0739/19/© 2019 Elsevier Inc. All rights reserved.

INTRODUCTION

Until the turn of the millennium, laminitis was largely considered a discrete disease entity with a common pathophysiology, regardless of the inciting cause. Ischemia was implicated as a primary mechanism, and, consequently, most modern research was focused on identifying the vascular events that caused laminitis, with therapeutic efforts in the clinic and the field largely designed to enhance digital perfusion, regardless of the underlying clinical scenario. However, the primary conditions that lead to laminitis are extremely diverse and, in many of these clinical situations, it is difficult to rationally attribute laminitis solely to ischemia of the hoof lamellae. New research began to focus on the lamellar epithelial cells and, in particular, their adhesions (both to other epithelial cells as well as to the extracellular matrix); armed with novel methods and technology, researchers were able to perform studies evaluating molecular events within the lamellae during the development of laminitis in different experimental models. Combined with work that focused for the first time on insulin dysregulation and its role in laminitis development, this research has led to the recognition in the last decade that there are key differences in the pathophysiology of laminitis that depend on the inciting cause. However, there is convergence in some mechanistic events during development of the laminitis lesion: at a molecular signaling level; in the nature and progression of adhesion failure within the lamellar epithelium; and in the response to injury, which seems to be similar regardless of the cause. The differences and similarities in the pathogenesis of different forms of laminitis have important implications for how clinicians rationally approach prevention and treatment of laminitis in different clinical situations.

WHAT IS LAMINITIS?

The term laminitis is used to describe the clinical and pathologic consequences of disturbances in the attachment between inner hoof wall and distal phalanx that is normally provided by the digital lamellae. Importantly, the lamellae normally act to suspend the bone within the hoof capsule, and it is the largely unrecoverable loss of this suspensory function that leads to the lameness, dysfunction, and morphologic derangements characteristic of chronic laminitis. However, laminitis can be surprisingly difficult to accurately define. Because it occurs secondary to a diverse range of primary diseases or conditions rather than on its own as a lone phenomenon, it cannot be considered a discrete disease. A recent review suggested that laminitis may be better described as a clinical syndrome[1]; however, laminitis commonly exists without overt clinical signs and therefore may also be viewed primarily as a lesion (an abnormal change in structure of an organ or tissue caused by injury or disease[2]), with characteristic gross and microscopic structural/ultrastructural changes as well as molecular events used to characterize it.

Because of the unique mechanical role of this tissue, essentially anything that disturbs homeostasis within the lamellae has the potential to cause attachment failure, secondary damage, and pain; this characteristic is perhaps most responsible for the diversity of primary conditions and situations that can lead to laminitis. Failure of the lamellar attachment can be attributed largely to a combination of:

1. Loss of the normal cell shape (stretching) of the lamellar epithelial cells
2. Failure of epithelial cell adhesions (both between cells and to the dermis via the basement membrane [BM]; **Fig. 1**)

The BM and other components of the extracellular matrix may also be variably damaged, weakening the attachment between epidermis and dermis. Resultant

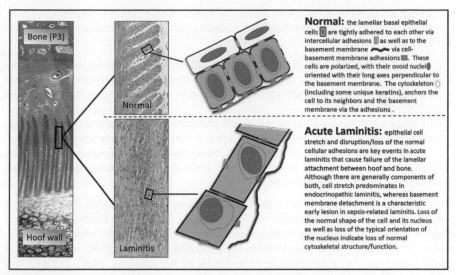

Normal: the lamellar basal epithelial cells ▊ are tightly adhered to each other via intercellular adhesions ▊ as well as to the basement membrane ⌒⌒ via cell-basement membrane adhesions ▉. These cells are polarized, with their ovoid nuclei● oriented with their long axes perpendicular to the basement membrane. The cytoskeleton ◌ (including some unique keratins), anchors the cell to its neighbors and the basement membrane via the adhesions .

Acute Laminitis: epithelial cell stretch and disruption/loss of the normal cellular adhesions are key events in acute laminitis that cause failure of the lamellar attachment between hoof and bone. Although there are generally components of both, cell stretch predominates in endocrinopathic laminitis, whereas basement membrane detachment is a characteristic early lesion in sepsis-related laminitis. Loss of the normal shape of the cell and its nucleus as well as loss of the typical orientation of the nucleus indicate loss of normal cytoskeletal structure/function.

Fig. 1. Adhesion loss and cellular stretch are key mechanisms occurring at the level of the lamellar epithelial cell that lead to lamellar attachment failure in acute laminitis.

pathologic alterations in the lamellae can be mild and insidious, with slow and progressive lengthening of lamellae caused by stretch and cellular proliferation (as in many cases of endocrinopathic laminitis) or may be characterized by rapid loss of tissue mechanical integrity caused by widespread cellular dysadhesion and cytoskeletal failure (more common in sepsis-related laminitis [SRL] and supporting-limb laminitis [SLL]). After damage to any or all of the components of the lamellar attachment, the progression of laminitis depends on:

1. The severity and distribution of this initial damage
2. The forces acting on the tissue caused by weight bearing

These forces are governed by body weight, locomotor activity, and the variation in mechanics between individual feet, as shown by the discrepant severity of laminitis in the forefeet versus hindfeet in naturally occurring and experimentally induced laminitis, caused by differential weight distribution (60% of body weight borne on the forelimbs, 40% on the hind) and not differences in the severity of other underlying processes.[3]

Once the suspensory function of the lamellae is compromised, the pain, morphologic derangement, and progression of digital disorder are largely consequences of novel mechanical forces now acting between the distal phalanx, sole, and ground surface, together with the proliferative and dysplastic response of the lamellar epidermis to injury. These processes are shared and similar regardless of the inciting cause. However, over the last decade, researchers have recognized that there are key differences (and some similarities) in the initial events that lead to laminitis depending on the inciting cause. A focus on these early events is leading to a better understanding of why laminitis occurs in different clinical situations and is helping to identify therapeutic targets.

WHAT ARE THE MAIN FORMS OF LAMINITIS, WHAT CLINICAL SITUATIONS CAUSE THEM, AND WHAT MODELS ARE USED TO STUDY THEM?

Many individual causes of laminitis have been identified; one publication lists 80 separate causes, predispositions, and pathways for laminitis, including evidence-based and anecdotal observations of causes as diverse as snake bite and ingestion of cold water.[4] Today, it is recognized that most cases fit into 3 general categories based on the underlying cause:

1. Endocrinopathic laminitis is associated with insulin dysregulation, which may be primary (equine metabolic syndrome), associated with pituitary pars intermedia dysfunction (PPID), or iatrogenic (secondary to exogenous corticosteroid administration).
2. SRL occurs in horses with systemic illness characterized by systemic inflammation, particularly in response to endotoxemia (eg, colitis, metritis, pneumonia).
3. SLL develops in horses with painful limb conditions such as fractures or synovial sepsis; this form primarily affects the limb contralateral to the primary injury, but often multiple limbs are affected.

The current knowledge of laminitis is based largely on discoveries made through developing and using experimental models (**Table 1**). The recent discovery that maintenance of high blood insulin concentrations can induce laminitis experimentally in healthy ponies and horses (euglycemic-hyperinsulinemic clamp [EHC] model)[5,6] has greatly improved the understanding of endocrinopathic laminitis, which is by far the most common clinical form. High blood insulin concentrations probably exert a direct effect on the lamellae, and therefore the severity and duration of hyperinsulinemic episodes govern the severity and progression of laminitis in naturally occurring clinical cases. Many field cases of endocrinopathic laminitis therefore involve insidious and slowly progressive laminitis as a result of repeated mild insults; however, there are also some acute severe episodes, particularly if exposed to pasture rich in nonstructural carbohydrates (NSCs). Although the EHC model reliably causes laminitis in experimental subjects, it does not mimic the natural development of endocrinopathic laminitis, being much more severe and acute than natural disease. The infusion of glucose alone (to produce an endogenous hyperinsulinemic response)[7] and feeding a high-NSC challenge diet to animals with insulin dysregulation[8] are emerging experimental models that may have more clinical relevance, particularly when testing interventions.

A source of major confusion in understanding laminitis is that the experimental model of choice for the induction of SRL is also the administration of excessive NSC in the form of alimentary carbohydrate overload. Either starch or oligofructose is administered as a large bolus, destined to transit to the hindgut and lead to rapid fermentation, gram-positive bacterial proliferation, and colitis (failure of the hindgut

Table 1
Major forms of laminitis and their corresponding experimental models

Type of Laminitis	Experimental Model
Sepsis-related laminitis	Black walnut extract model[10]
	Enteral carbohydrate overload model
	• Wood/corn starch model[3]
	• Oligofructose model[10]
Endocrinopathic laminitis	Euglycemic-hyperinsulinemic clamp[5]
	Glucose infusion model[7]
	NSC challenge diet in horses with insulin dysregulation[8]
Supporting limb laminitis	Modified shoe to cause uneven weight bearing[14]

Abbreviation: NSC, nonstructural carbohydrates.

mucosal barrier and absorption of substances including endotoxin). In contrast with more modest dietary challenges with NSC designed to invoke a hyperinsulinemic response in predisposed animals, carbohydrate overload models cause endotoxemia and systemic inflammation reminiscent of naturally occurring colitis.[9] It is unclear why alimentary carbohydrate overload is such a reliable cause of acute laminitis: greater than 90% of horses dosed with oligofructose develop laminitis[10] compared with 25% to 30% of clinical colitis cases.[11] The enhanced effects of carbohydrate overload do not seem to be caused by a concurrent hyperinsulinemic response, which does not occur with oligofructose overload.[12,13] A model for the study of SLL has recently been developed using a shoe insert that induces nonpainful preferential weight bearing in a forelimb[14]; however, this model lacks several elements that are often present in clinical cases of SLL (pain, stress, and components of inflammation caused by tissue damage associated with the primary injury or secondary infection).

IS THE LESION CONSISTENT REGARDLESS OF THE INCITING CAUSE?

Experimental studies provide the opportunity to evaluate early developmental lesions; however, there are no published direct comparisons between different forms of laminitis that focus on these preclinical lesions. Studies of naturally occurring laminitis cases, by their very nature, are limited to more advanced acute and chronic lesions. Regardless, experimental studies show that the lamellar epithelial cell is central to the initial events that lead to initial lamellar failure in all 3 major forms of laminitis through a combination of loss of the normal cell shape (stretching) of the lamellar epithelial cells and failure of epithelial cell adhesions (both between cells and to the dermis via the BM). In experimental endocrinopathic laminitis, epithelial cell stretch seems to contribute to initial lengthening of secondary epidermal lamellae (SEL), preceding cellular proliferation and BM dysadhesion,[15] whereas, in SRL, BM detachment and inflammatory changes (leukocyte infiltration) seem to be key early events.[16,17] Direct comparison of lesions in the acute phase (after the onset of lameness) in models of SRL and endocrinopathic laminitis reveal common components, including lengthening and narrowing of SEL, rounding and disorientation of lamellar epithelial cell nuclei, and increased mitosis and apoptosis (accelerated cell death/proliferation cycle).[18] Although evidence of inflammation and BM detachment have been considered to be less prominent with EHC laminitis, there seems to be considerable variation between studies, with a recent EHC study in Standardbred horses revealing the presence of severe BM detachment and leukocyte infiltration similar to that observed in sepsis models at a similar time point.[19] It is possible that variations in the acuteness/rate of lesion progression are responsible for the discrepancy in appearance of lesions between the different forms of laminitis (both experimental and naturally occurring) rather than differences in the underlying cellular processes at work. Similarly, the influence of distraction caused by weight bearing plays a critical role in the progression of the lesion, and it can be difficult to determine what elements of the lesion are purely consequences of this factor. This difficulty is shown by differences in the severity and nature of forelimb and hind limb lesions in both endocrinopathic laminitis and SRL[3] and also between ponies and light-breed horses in endocrinopathic lamintiis.[6,20] Lesions in ponies subjected to hyperinsulinemia (even in the acute phase) are characterized by SEL lengthening caused by cell stretch (rather than being caused by proliferation) with little to no BM detachment or inflammation.[21]

Regardless of the inciting cause, the progression of the laminitis lesion after the acute phase seems to share common elements characteristic of an epithelial wound healing response, with dysplastic epithelial cell proliferation and dyskeratosis.[18,21–25] A similar pattern is evident even after a traumatic event such as after biopsy of the lamellae, highlighting the limited nature of the lamellar epithelial response to injury (**Fig. 2**).

WHAT ARE THE IMPORTANT UNDERLYING MECHANISMS THAT LEAD TO DIFFERENT FORMS OF LAMINITIS?

Although there has been great effort focused on identifying a single common pathway through which diverse systemic conditions might lead to lamellar dysfunction and failure, it is more likely that the reason such diverse entities cause laminitis is that any insult to the lamellar epithelial cells has the potential to disrupt the highly differentiated, polarized nature of the lamellar epithelial cells and thus their cytoskeletal and adhesion complex dynamics. In turn, the unique mechanical stresses on these cells under normal conditions mean that even minor insults can result in cell stretch and/or loss of adhesion and therefore lamellar attachment failure. Through epidemiologic and experimental studies, important factors and processes relevant to each form of laminitis with the potential to disrupt lamellar homeostasis are gradually being identified (**Fig. 3**).

ENDOCRINOPATHIC LAMINITIS

Endocrinopathic laminitis is now reported to be the most common form of the disease, affecting primarily equids with a phenotype of obesity (especially regional adiposity)

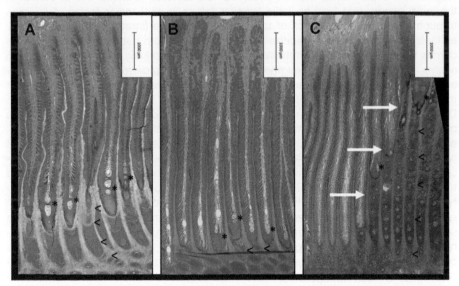

Fig. 2. The proliferative dysplastic epithelial healing response is similar regardless of the inciting cause of laminitis. Sections of early chronic endocrinopathic laminitis (*A*). There is widespread distortion, fusion, and thickening of the SEL, with epithelial proliferation and dyskeratosis. In the abaxial region (toward the hoof wall; bottom of the image) marked lamellar dysplasia with merging/bridging of the lamellae and hyperkeratosis is noted (*asterisks*) along with the formation of abnormal new keratinized tissue (so-called cap horn; *arrowheads*), contributing to the lamellar wedge. Similar changes are present in the section from a subacute SRL case (*B*), although they are more pronounced axially, perhaps because of severe separation in this region during the acute insult. Trauma causes a similar healing response (*C*) to laminitis: in this case a biopsy of the lamellae had been harvested from this site (*arrows*) 12 months before obtaining this section (H&E, original magnification ×10). (*Courtesy of* Dr Julie Engiles [*A*].)

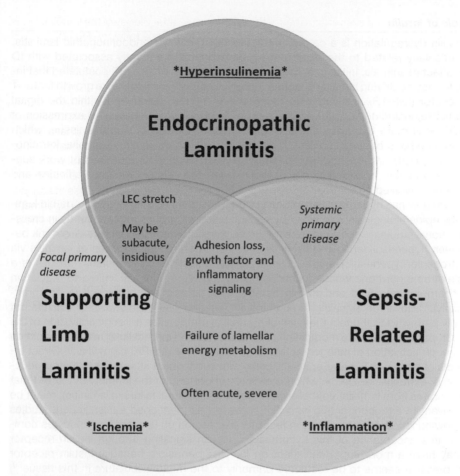

Fig. 3. Common and unique mechanisms for the 3 major clinical forms of laminitis. LEC, lamellar epithelial cell.

and insulin dysregulation (ID), particularly when they are exposed to a diet containing abundant nonstructural carbohydrate (NSC).[26–28] Clinical observations and the results of epidemiologic studies have suggested that the risk of endocrinopathic laminitis is heightened when equids graze pastures with high NSC content (ie, fructans, monosaccharides, and/or starch), and theories on the pathogenesis of laminitis in this setting have been extrapolated from experimental models of enteral carbohydrate overload (such as wood/corn starch and oligofructose administration). However, the extent to which these severe experimental carbohydrate overload models reflect events occurring during the development of laminitis related to ID is questionable. It is likely that the amount and rate of starch or fructan administered for induction of carbohydrate overload in these studies far exceeds the quantity of NSC ingested by grazing equids (at least over a short period of time; as with laminitis lesion development, rate of administration/intake seems to be important). In addition, previous experimental studies have not used animals with a phenotype typically associated with risk of endocrinopathic laminitis (eg, overweight, predisposed breed) and thus have not addressed the likely interaction between diet and phenotypic factors associated with laminitis susceptibility.

Role of Insulin

Insulin dysregulation is a central predictive risk factor for endocrinopathic laminitis, particularly related to the persistent hyperinsulinemia frequently associated with ID in affected animals. Initial hypotheses generated based on this risk postulated that insulin may be driving lamellar changes through its affinity for insulin-like growth factor-1 receptor (IGF-1R). Insulin's own receptor has limited distribution within the digital lamellae, including very little expression by keratinocytes[29]; however, expression of IGF-1R is more extensive and abundant than insulin receptor in this tissue, which could perhaps be a mechanism through which insulin could signal lamellar keratinocytes directly and change their phenotype. That being said, more recent work suggests that this is exceptionally unlikely, given the relative receptor affinities and kinetics involved.[30]

Not only has hyperinsulinemia been strongly associated with endocrinopathic laminitis epidemiologically (identified by several research groups independently in cross-sectional studies[27,31,32]), but recent studies have characterized a more direct link between hyperinsulinemia and laminitis with the experimental induction of laminitis via iatrogenic hyperinsulinemia in normal ponies[5] and light-breed horses.[6] Insulin is a pleiotropic hormone whose functions historically were primarily limited to regulation of carbohydrate, lipid, and protein metabolism in times of energy excess (ie, postprandially).[33] However, signaling through insulin receptor has been shown to activate not only pathways that direct the fates of nutritional metabolites (through activation of the PI3K pathway) but also modulation of mitogenesis and extracellular matrix production through activation of mitogen-activated protein kinase (MAPK) pathways.[34] Direct effects of insulin on lamellar epithelial cells, with subsequent alterations in their production of extracellular matrix (which is critically important for the integrity of the BM that separates from lamellar epithelial cells, defining structural failure in laminitis), might be relevant to endocrinopathic laminitis. However, as mentioned earlier, recent studies showing little evidence of insulin receptor expression on lamellar keratinocytes complicates acceptance of this hypothesis.[29] Insulin signaling through insulin receptor may have a more important effect on lamellar perfusion, because insulin receptor expression seems to be restricted primarily to the microvasculature in this tissue[29]; however, little evidence exists to support a microvascular perfusion deficit in the setting of acute endocrinopathic laminitis (van Eps, unpublished data, 2019). Importantly, activation of insulin receptor or IGF-1R can promote signaling through the mammalian target of rapamycin (mTOR) pathway, directly linking energy metabolism and response to nutritional substrate with regulation of cytoskeletal elements and epithelial differentiation.[35] This link may represent an attractive target for therapy and prevention of this disease, and further investigation is needed.

Role of Glucose

Glucose is an important energy source for cells of the equine digital lamellae and supports the structural integrity of this tissue; severe glucose deprivation has been shown ex vivo to be associated with lamellar failure.[36] However, glucose uptake within the lamellae does not seem to be insulin dependent. Glucose promotes inflammatory signaling, it can drive/support epithelial-to-mesenchymal transition in epithelial cells, and it is present in abundance in the EHC model of endocrinopathic laminitis. Although ID and subsequent glucose starvation have been suggested in the past as potential mechanisms that might cause lamellar dysfunction, it has been shown[37] that the primary glucose transporter (GLUT) type expressed in laminae is GLUT1, which is neither insulin dependent nor highly insulin responsive (such as the GLUT4 transporter, which is more abundant in skeletal muscle, liver, and adipose tissue). So, instead of glucose deprivation in the setting of ID, the digital lamellae may experience an increased glucose flux in the setting of ID. The significance of this remains to be determined, but, given the potential molecular effects of glucotoxicity that have been shown to occur in other tissues, it seems important to further clarify its role in the setting of endocrinopathic laminitis.

Role of Leptin

Leptin is an adipokine hormone expressed primarily in white adipose tissue, and its concentrations in peripheral blood from horses have been shown to correlate well with the degree of adiposity of the animal. Although leptin (along with insulin) has also been identified in some epidemiologic studies of horses as a risk factor for endocrinopathic laminitis,[26] its role in the pathophysiology of laminitis has not been investigated thoroughly. Leptin has been shown to significantly alter the physiology and differentiation of epithelial cells (including keratinocytes) in other species both in vivo and in vitro,[38] and leptin can independently stimulate dysadhesion of epithelial cells from neighboring cells and their BM, encouraging adoption of a more mesenchymal phenotype (ie, epithelial-mesenchymal transition [EMT]).[39] If these changes were to occur within the equine digital lamellae, the end result could be lamellar failure. Obese horses are consistently hyperleptinemic,[40–42] and further investigation of the role of leptin in normal digital lamellar physiology and the pathophysiology of endocrinopathic laminitis is needed.

SEPSIS-RELATED LAMINITIS

Laminitis is a common consequence of diseases complicated by the systemic inflammatory response syndrome, particularly when gram-negative bacterial infection or bacterial products (including endotoxin) are driving this inflammatory response (sepsis). In a recent retrospective study, clinical evidence of sepsis/endotoxemia was confirmed as a risk factor for the development of laminitis.[43] Sepsis is differentiated from simple infection by the presence of an aberrant or dysregulated host response (inflammatory, coagulopathic, and metabolic derangements) and organ dysfunction.[44] The development of end-organ dysfunction (multiple organ dysfunction syndrome [MODS]) has a major effect on survival in humans with sepsis, and similarly laminitis seems to be a form of end-organ dysfunction with critical importance to survival for adult horses with sepsis. However, the pathophysiology of MODS (and sepsis-associated laminitis) is still poorly understood. Research has focused on mechanisms that could disrupt cellular homeostasis in sepsis, including circulatory derangements, inflammatory processes, apoptosis, and derangements of cellular energy metabolism.

Perfusion and Energy Balance

Although there is some evidence of microvascular dysfunction in MODS and laminitis, there is no compelling evidence of ischemia during laminitis development.[45] Disturbances of energy metabolism despite adequate perfusion have been increasingly recognized in the pathophysiology of human sepsis-related organ failure[46–51] and involve primarily mitochondrial dysfunction/dysregulation but also dysregulation of glycolysis and lipid metabolism. Although energy stress did not seem to feature early in laminitis development in a sepsis-related (oligofructose) model, there is some limited evidence of nonischemic oxidative energy failure early in acute laminitis in this same model; however, this may be a secondary event.[52]

Role of Inflammation

The central role of inflammation in the pathogenesis of acute laminitis has been highlighted experimentally, with endothelial activation, cytokine and chemokine upregulation, and leukocyte emigration into the lamellar tissue occurring early during the development of experimentally induced laminitis.[53–57] There is little evidence that apoptosis or oxidative damage play a primary role in laminitis development.[58,59]

Extracellular Matrix Degradation

Because the lamellae have a unique mechanical support role, the lamellar epithelial cell adhesions and the integrity of the extracellular matrix have received special research attention. Recent evidence suggests that degradation of extracellular matrix components by matrix metalloproteinase enzymes seems to play only a secondary role.[60,61]

Other Factors

Although ID may be a feature of sepsis in horses,[62] it is clear from experimental SRL models using carbohydrate overload[9,10,63] that laminitis develops in the absence of clinically significant hyperinsulinemia. However, the exact pathways leading from the systemic inflammation of sepsis to lamellar structural failure remain unclear.

SUPPORTING-LIMB LAMINITIS

SLL remains a primary limiting factor to long-term treatment success in horses with painful limb conditions, including fractures. The onset of SLL is unpredictable and once clinically apparent it tends to be rapidly progressive. The incidence has been estimated at approximately 10% to 15% of horses that present for painful limb problems (or require limb casts) in North American studies, with body weight and duration of casting identified as risk factors in 1 study.[64–67] Mechanical and vascular mechanisms have been considered by investigators as potential contributors to the pathophysiology of SLL, but there is very little published evidence.[65,68]

Mechanical Factors

It is well accepted that, in standing horses, the body mass is divided between the forelimbs and hindlimbs approximately in a 60:40 ratio[69]; therefore, a single forelimb is subjected to vertical ground reaction forces equivalent to approximately 0.3 times body weight in a square stance. Peak ground reaction forces on a single limb increase to be equivalent to greater than 0.5 times body weight at the walk, 1.2 times body weight at the trot, and up to 3 times body weight at the gallop, and therefore it seems unlikely that compensatory load redistribution in a standing horse could exceed the mechanical tensile strength of the lamellae. However, consistent increases in load (even if modest) could potentially trigger lamellar epidermal remodeling: there is existing evidence that such remodeling occurs in response to mechanical stresses associated with normal locomotion,[70–73] and this has important implications for the pathophysiology of SLL.

Perfusion and Energy Balance

There is growing evidence that cyclic limb loading is critical for normal lamellar perfusion and that perfusion deficits and negative energy balance contribute to the development of SLL. Maintenance of lamellar epithelial adhesions required to withstand immense mechanical stress is an energy-consuming process; therefore, glucose consumption by the digit is high and uptake is non–insulin dependent (GLUT-1 transporter mediated) in the lamellae.[37,74] There is no means for local glycogen storage, so uptake must be matched by constant delivery via the blood. Despite this, the normal lamellar dermis (responsible for nutrient and oxygen delivery to the lamellar epithelial cells) is poorly perfused[75] and hypoxic.[76] Glucose deprivation in vitro causes disruption of lamellar epithelial adhesion and cytoskeletal dynamics and loss of lamellar structural integrity.[36,77] Imaging studies have shown that limb load affects digital perfusion,[68,78,79] and studies show that lamellar perfusion and energy balance depend on limb load cycling (weight shifting/walking).[45,80] A recent study using a preferential weight-bearing model showed increases in lamellar hypoxia-inducible factor 1α concentration in the supporting-limb lamellae in the absence of changes in inflammatory signaling, supporting a role for ischemia in the development of SLL,[14] and studies using this model are ongoing.

Other Factors

The contribution of other factors, such as systemic inflammation and endocrine dysregulation (implicated in other forms of laminitis), to the development of SLL remains unclear; however, many SLL cases in clinical practice are complicated by infection and presumably have at least transient periods of ID during treatment of their primary injury,[65] and this warrants further study.

WHAT MECHANISMS ARE SHARED BETWEEN DIFFERENT FORMS?

Whether or not there are common mechanistic pathways for different forms of laminitis may be largely a question of timing. Although the initial events suspected to cause disruption of lamellar epithelial cell homeostasis seem to be different, the end result is the same: lamellar epithelial cell stretch and adhesion failure, leading to failure of the suspensory function of the lamellae with secondary trauma caused by distractive forces acting on the weakened tissue. These distractive forces, associated with weight bearing and ambulation (and therefore dependent on body weight and locomotor activity), are a common element in all cases and have a major influence on lesion progression. Subsequent inflammation, pain, and a proliferative epithelial wound response are also common pathophysiologic elements in all cases. Inflammation can be assumed to be an important common event in acute laminitis regardless of cause and is an initial contributor to pain, another major shared element of laminitis pathophysiology. Pain has a complex pathogenesis in laminitis and its primary sources vary with the chronicity of the laminitis. Rather than being a mere secondary consequence, pain may also contribute to disease pathogenesis: in a rodent fracture model, remote paw epithelial proliferation was attributed to neurogenic signaling caused by pain, mediated through substance P.[81] Although that has not been shown in horses, morphologic and molecular changes typical of neuropathic pain states are found in the digital nerves of horses with chronic laminitis, showing that pain may be an active contributor to disease progression in laminitis, and this warrants further investigation.[82]

The proliferative, dysplastic, and dyskeratotic response of the lamellar epithelium is common to all forms of laminitis and eventually leads to formation of the characteristic lamellar wedge.[83] However, there is also evidence of increased epithelial cell proliferation early in acute experimental endocrinopathic laminitis, observed as an accelerated apoptosis-proliferation cycle in tissue from ponies undergoing the EHC.[21] The authors have also observed an early proliferative response in the preferential weight-bearing model (Andrew van Eps, unpublished data, 2019) and there is a clear proliferative response after acute experimental SRL.[24] It may seem rational that epithelial cell proliferation is the cause of lamellar dysadhesion; however, epithelial cell stretch and adhesion loss seem to precede the proliferative response in experimental studies. Dissolution of adhesions and cytoskeletal rearrangement are key events in cells undergoing epithelial-mesenchymal transition in disease processes, including cancer,[84,85] and are triggered by signaling through the central mTORC1 pathway. Activation of mTORC1 signaling in lamellae has recently been shown in 2 models of endocrinopathic laminitis,[86] and the authors have preliminary evidence indicating similar activation in models of SRL and SLL, suggesting it may be a common pathway in all forms (Teresa Burns, unpublished data, 2019). Increased concentrations of energy substrates (glucose, amino acids), activation of growth factor signaling (eg, IGF-1), and decreased activation of metabolic counter-regulatory enzymes (such as AMP-activated protein kinase [AMPK]) can all result in activation of mTOR signaling (and all may be relevant at various times during the pathogenesis of the different forms of laminitis). Further research is needed to determine the importance of this pathway to lesion development and whether it represents a therapeutic target.

WHAT ARE THE IMPLICATIONS FOR PREVENTION AND TREATMENT IN THE CLINIC?

Based on this current knowledge of major mechanisms, preventive and early therapeutic efforts should be aimed at:

- Perfusion enhancement in horses at risk of SLL
- Control of local and systemic inflammation for SRL
- Early diagnosis and careful management of ID for endocrinopathic laminitis

Treatment regimens that address these specific aspects of the underlying cause but also follow principles that are common regardless of the inciting cause are more likely to lead to favorable outcomes (**Fig. 4**).

Perfusion Enhancement for Supporting-limb Laminitis

It seems that cyclic loading and unloading of the feet plays an essential role in maintaining normal lamellar microvascular perfusion. The key to SLL prevention is therefore likely to be the development of strategies to monitor and then regulate limb load cycling frequency in the supporting limbs of patients at risk. Monitoring should include some form of serial assessment of limb load cycling activity: a method that can detect both walking steps as well as more subtle weight-shifting events requires development and validation. In horses at risk, regular encouragement to walk may be beneficial; however, there are insufficient data to support specific recommendations at this stage, and the logistics of this intervention may depend on the nature and severity of the primary condition. Strategies to reduce load on the supporting limb may include partial (and preferably dynamic) sling support and perhaps even periodic forced recumbency.[87] Careful attention to analgesia for the primary condition will help to normalize limb weight distribution and cycling frequency; however, medications with a sedative effect may be best avoided. Although sedation may help to encourage recumbency, it also reduces voluntary exercise and limb load cycling in stabled patients and therefore may be contraindicated in these cases.

Controlling Systemic and Local Inflammation in Sepsis-related Laminitis

Therapeutic efforts to control the primary disease and systemic inflammation in cases of equine sepsis are paramount. Intravenous fluids for circulatory support, binding of circulating endotoxin using polymyxin B, and hyperimmune plasma and the use of nonsteroidal antiinflammatory drugs to control downstream inflammation are

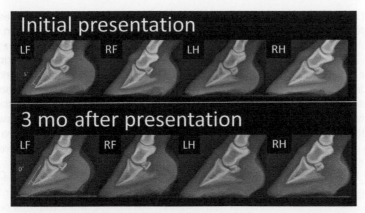

Fig. 4. Forelimb and hind limb foot radiographs from a 3-year-old Welsh pony gelding at presentation (*above*): the pony developed signs of acute laminitis after access to lush pasture. Initial treatment included continuous digital hypothermia, phenylbutazone, and impression material orthotics. Despite normal body condition, an oral sugar test was performed revealing a marked hyperinsulinemic response (>500 mU/L) to ingested sugar, so treatment with oral metformin was initiated and strict dietary control implemented. The pony regained soundness after 7 days. Repeat radiographic evaluation revealed clear resolution of dorsopalmar/plantar rotation within 3 months (*below*). Although a low body weight was advantageous in this case, the resolution of radiographic changes shows that some reversal of laminitis may be possible with early, aggressive therapy that uses rational first aid strategies and (most importantly) targets the underlying primary cause (ID in this case). LF, left fore; LH, left hind; RF, right fore; RH, right hind.

reasonable treatment strategies, particularly in cases of sepsis associated with gastrointestinal disease.[88] Although 1 study seemed to identify a possible protective effect of low-molecular-weight heparin in surgical colic cases, the control group was historical and the evidence weak.[89] Treatment with unfractionated heparin failed to influence the development of sepsis-related laminitis induced experimentally with carbohydrate overload.[90] Continuous digital hypothermia (cryotherapy) has a marked antiinflammatory effect in experimental models of SRL,[91] and there is evidence that hypothermia is a clinically effective prophylactic strategy for the prevention of laminitis in horses with colitis.[11]

Controlling Insulin Dysregulation in Endocrinopathic Laminitis

Strategies to minimize serum insulin concentrations over time are thought to be central to prevention and treatment of endocrinopathic laminitis. To this end, techniques that minimize increases in blood glucose concentration and therefore the exaggerated acute insulin response to glucose in these animals should be helpful; examples include minimizing dietary NSC content (a commonly recommended target is <10% on a dry matter basis for all dietary components) and possibly using sodium-glucose cotransporter-2 inhibitors such as velagliflozin[8] to encourage glycosuria and decrease blood sugar levels. Pharmacologic interventions that enhance systemic insulin sensitivity/responsiveness would also be beneficial, because they should in theory enhance postprandial glucose disposal and minimize its effects on pancreatic insulin secretion. Regular aerobic exercise (as long as orthopedic pain/instability does not preclude it) should also improve systemic insulin and glucose dynamics, even in the absence of weight loss, and should be encouraged as much as possible.[92] Early diagnosis and control of underlying PPID that may be driving ID is also critical in these cases. Drugs and nutraceuticals that act as functional AMPK mimetics (such as metformin, resveratrol, aspirin, bitter melon, green tea catechin, and curcumin) or inhibitors of mTOR signaling may act both to improve systemic insulin and glucose dynamics and to improve epithelial differentiation and polarity (and thereby counteract influences that tend to drive an epithelial-to-mesenchymal transition); although these effects have been reasonably well documented in other species,[93–95] they remain to be described similarly well in horses. Inhibition of cyclooxegenase-2, which has been shown to be upregulated in lamellar tissue in diverse models of laminitis[57,96] and to drive EMT,[97] may also complement novel treatment and prevention strategies in the future.

Common Treatment Principles for Acute Laminitis Regardless of the Inciting Cause

In acute laminitis cases the aims should be:

- Aggressive treatment of the underlying condition
- Minimization of further lamellar damage
- Provision of analgesia
- Monitoring of progression

Aggressive and early control of ID (using diet as well as medications such as metformin if necessary) is critical in acute endocrinopathic cases.

Strategies to minimize ongoing lamellar damage include:

- Antiinflammatory therapy
- Confinement and restriction of locomotor activity
- Mechanical foot support
- Digital hypothermia

The influence of mechanical distraction on outcome cannot be overemphasized: every effort should be made to minimize this in acute cases while the strength of the lamellar attachment is compromised. Restriction of ambulation is paramount, and horses should be confined to a stall and encouraged to lie down by providing deep comfortable bedding. Tranquillizers and sedatives may encourage recumbency and reduce voluntary ambulation in horses with acute laminitis. Further minimization of distractive forces can be achieved by redistribution of load from the hoof wall onto the frog/caudal sole and facilitation of breakover using conservative trimming, orthotic support material, and/or bedding material (eg, sand).

Continuous digital hypothermia is the only therapy that has been shown to alter the progression of acute laminitis lesions. The application of digital hypothermia in acute SRL (even after lameness develops) limits lesion progression.[98] There is also new evidence showing a preventive effect in the hyperinsulinemic clamp model of endocrinopathic laminitis, suggesting that effects on common mechanistic events (inflammation, growth factor signaling) may be most important therapeutically. This finding also provides rationale for the use of hypothermia as a first aid measure in cases of endocrinopathic laminitis as well as SRL.

SUMMARY

Current evidence suggests that there are pathophysiologic factors that are unique to each form of laminitis but also common elements in both the developmental and acute stages of laminitis. The clinical implications are that clinicians can now use this information to formulate more precise preventive and therapeutic plans tailored to individual cases, which will undoubtedly improve clinical outcomes.

REFERENCES

1. Patterson-Kane JC, Karikoski NP, McGowan CM. Paradigm shifts in understanding equine laminitis. Vet J 2018;231:33–40.
2. Lesion [def. 2]. (n.d.). in Merriam Webster online. Available at: http://Www. merriam-webster.com/dictionary/lesion?utm_campaign=sd&utm_medium=serp &utm_source=jsonld. Accessed February 22, 2019.
3. Leise BS, Faleiros RR, Watts M, et al. Hindlimb laminar inflammatory response is similar to that present in forelimbs after carbohydrate overload in horses. Equine Vet J 2012;44(6):633–9.
4. Heymering HW. 80 causes, predispositions, and pathways of laminitis. Vet Clin North Am Equine Pract 2010;26:13–9.
5. Asplin KE, Sillence MN, Pollitt CC, et al. Induction of laminitis by prolonged hyperinsulinaemia in clinically normal ponies. Vet J 2007;174(3):530–5.
6. de Laat MA, McGowan CM, Sillence MN, et al. Equine laminitis: Induced by 48 h hyperinsulinaemia in standardbred horses. Equine Vet J 2010;42(2):129–35.
7. de Laat MA, Sillence MN, McGowan CM, et al. Continuous intravenous infusion of glucose induces endogenous hyperinsulinaemia and lamellar histopathology in standardbred horses. Vet J 2012;191(3):317–22.
8. Meier A, Reiche D, de Laat M, et al. The sodium-glucose co-transporter 2 inhibitor velagliflozin reduces hyperinsulinemia and prevents laminitis in insulin-dysregulated ponies. PLoS One 2018;13(9):e0203655.
9. Pollitt CC, Visser MB. Carbohydrate alimentary overload laminitis. Vet Clin North Am Equine Pract 2010;26(1):65–78.
10. van Eps AW, Pollitt CC. Equine laminitis induced with oligofructose. Equine Vet J 2006;38(3):203–8.
11. Kullman A, Holcombe SJ, Hurcombe SD, et al. Prophylactic digital cryotherapy is associated with decreased incidence of laminitis in horses diagnosed with colitis. Equine Vet J 2013;46(5):554–9.
12. Kalck KA, Frank N, Elliott SB, et al. Effects of low-dose oligofructose treatment administered via nasogastric intubation on induction of laminitis and associated alterations in glucose and insulin dynamics in horses. Am J Vet Res 2009; 70(5):624–32.
13. Toth F, Frank N, Elliott SB, et al. Effects of an intravenous endotoxin challenge on glucose and insulin dynamics in horses. Am J Vet Res 2008;69(1):82–8.
14. Gardner AK, van Eps AW, Watts MR, et al. A novel model to assess lamellar signaling relevant to preferential weight bearing in the horse. Vet J 2017;221: 62–7.
15. de Laat MA, Patterson-Kane JC, Pollitt CC, et al. Histological and morphometric lesions in the pre-clinical, developmental phase of insulin-induced laminitis in standardbred horses. Vet J 2013;195(3):305–12.
16. Visser MB, Pollitt CC. Lamellar leukocyte infiltration and involvement of IL-6 during oligofructose-induced equine laminitis development. Vet Immunol Immunopathol 2011;144(1–2):120–8.
17. Visser MB, Pollitt CC. The timeline of lamellar basement membrane changes during equine laminitis development. Equine Vet J 2011;43:471–7.
18. de Laat MA, van Eps AW, McGowan CM, et al. Equine laminitis: Comparative histopathology 48 hours after experimental induction with insulin or alimentary oligofructose in standardbred horses. J Comp Pathol 2011;145(4):399–409.

19. Stokes SM, Belknap JK, Engiles JB, et al. Continuous digital hypothermia prevents lamellar failure in the euglycaemic hyperinsulinemic clamp model of equine laminitis. Equine Vet J 2019. [Epub ahead of print].
20. Asplin KE, Patterson-Kane JC, Sillence MN, et al. Histopathology of insulin-induced laminitis in ponies. Equine Vet J 2010;42(8):700–6.
21. Karikoski NP, Patterson-Kane JC, Asplin KE, et al. Morphological and cellular changes in secondary epidermal lamellae of horses with insulin-induced laminitis. Am J Vet Res 2014;75(2):161–8.
22. Karikoski NP, McGowan CM, Singer ER, et al. Pathology of natural cases of equine endocrinopathic laminitis associated with hyperinsulinemia. Vet Pathol 2015;52(5):945–56.
23. Karikoski NP, Patterson-Kane JC, Singer ER, et al. Lamellar pathology in horses with pituitary pars intermedia dysfunction. Equine Vet J 2016;48(4):472–8.
24. Van Eps AW, Pollitt CC. Equine laminitis model: lamellar histopathology seven days after induction with oligofructose. Equine Vet J 2009;41(8):735–40.
25. Engiles JB, Galantino-Homer HL, Boston R, et al. Osteopathology in the equine distal phalanx associated with the development and progression of laminitis. Vet Pathol 2015;52(5):928–44.
26. Carter RA, Treiber KH, Geor RJ, et al. Prediction of incipient pasture-associated laminitis from hyperinsulinaemia, hyperleptinaemia and generalised and localised obesity in a cohort of ponies. Equine Vet J 2009;41(2):171–8.
27. Treiber KH, Kronfeld DS, Hess TM, et al. Evaluation of genetic and metabolic predispositions and nutritional risk factors for pasture-associated laminitis in ponies. J Am Vet Med Assoc 2006;228(10):1538–45.
28. USDA-NAHMS. Lameness and laminitis in US horses. United States Department of Agriculture National Animal Health Monitoring System; 2000 (#N318.0400).
29. Burns TA, Watts MR, Weber PS, et al. Distribution of insulin receptor and insulin-like growth factor-1 receptor in the digital laminae of mixed-breed ponies: an immunohistochemical study. Equine Vet J 2012;45(3):326–32.
30. Nanayakkara SN, Rahnama S, Harris PA, et al. Characterization of insulin and IGF-1 receptor binding in equine liver and lamellar tissue: Implications for endocrinopathic laminitis. Domest Anim Endocrinol 2019;66:21–6.
31. Frank N, Elliott SB, Brandt LE, et al. Physical characteristics, blood hormone concentrations, and plasma lipid concentrations in obese horses with insulin resistance. J Am Vet Med Assoc 2006;228(9):1383–90.
32. Kronfeld DS, Treiber KH, Hess TM, et al. Metabolic syndrome in healthy ponies facilitates nutritional countermeasures against pasture laminitis. J Nutr 2006; 136(7 Suppl):2090S–3S.
33. Rask-Madsen C, Kahn CR. Tissue-specific insulin signaling, metabolic syndrome, and cardiovascular disease. Arterioscler Thromb Vasc Biol 2012;32(9): 2052–9.
34. Vigneri R, Squatrito S, Sciacca L. Insulin and its analogs: actions via insulin and IGF receptors. Acta Diabetol 2010;47(4):271–8.
35. Lane H, Geor RJ, Burns TA, et al. Laminar IGF-1 receptor signaling in a model of endocrinopathic laminitis. Proceedings of the Forum of the American College of Veterinary Internal Medicine. 2013.
36. Pass MA, Pollitt S, Pollitt CC. Decreased glucose metabolism causes separation of hoof lamellae in vitro: a trigger for laminitis? Equine Vet J Suppl 1998;(26): 133–8.
37. Asplin KE, Curlewis JD, McGowan CM, et al. Glucose transport in the equine hoof. Equine Vet J 2011;43(2):196–201.

38. Lee M, Lee E, Jin SH, et al. Leptin regulates the pro-inflammatory response in human epidermal keratinocytes. Arch Dermatol Res 2018;310(4):351–62.

39. Gui X, Chen H, Cai H, et al. Leptin promotes pulmonary fibrosis development by inhibiting autophagy via PI3K/akt/mTOR pathway. Biochem Biophys Res Commun 2018;498(3):660–6.

40. Schultz N, Geor RJ, Manfredi JM. Factors associated with leptin and adiponectin concentrations in a large across breed cohort of horses and ponies. J Vet Intern Med 2014;28:998.

41. Caltabilota TJ, Earl LR, Thompson DL Jr, et al. Hyperleptinemia in mares and geldings: assessment of insulin sensitivity from glucose responses to insulin injection. J Anim Sci 2010;88(9):2940–9.

42. Carter RA, McCutcheon LJ, Valle E, et al. Effects of exercise training on adiposity, insulin sensitivity, and plasma hormone and lipid concentrations in overweight or obese, insulin-resistant horses. Am J Vet Res 2010;71(3):314–21.

43. Parsons CS, Orsini JA, Krafty R, et al. Risk factors for development of acute laminitis in horses during hospitalization: 73 cases (1997-2004). J Am Vet Med Assoc 2007;230(6):885–9.

44. Singer M, Deutschman CS, Seymour CW, et al. The third international consensus definitions for sepsis and septic shock (sepsis-3). JAMA 2016;315(8):801–10.

45. Medina-Torres CE, Underwood C, Pollitt CC, et al. Microdialysis measurements of equine lamellar perfusion and energy metabolism in response to physical and pharmacological manipulations of blood flow. Equine Vet J 2016;48(6):756–64.

46. Arulkumaran N, Deutschman CS, Pinsky MR, et al. Mitochondrial function in sepsis. Shock 2016;45(3):271–81.

47. Arulkumaran N, Pollen S, Greco E, et al. Renal tubular cell mitochondrial dysfunction occurs despite preserved renal oxygen delivery in experimental septic acute kidney injury. Crit Care Med 2018;46(4):e318–25.

48. Kao C, Hsu J, Bandi V, et al. Alterations in glutamine metabolism and its conversion to citrulline in sepsis. Am J Physiol Endocrinol Metab 2013;304(12): E1359–64.

49. Trentadue R, Fiore F, Massaro F, et al. Induction of mitochondrial dysfunction and oxidative stress in human fibroblast cultures exposed to serum from septic patients. Life Sci 2012;91(7–8):237–43.

50. Mantzarlis K, Tsolaki V, Zakynthinos E. Role of oxidative stress and mitochondrial dysfunction in sepsis and potential therapies. Oxid Med Cell Longev 2017;2017: 5985209.

51. Hansen ME, Simmons KJ, Tippetts TS, et al. Lipopolysaccharide disrupts mitochondrial physiology in skeletal muscle via disparate effects on sphingolipid metabolism. Shock 2015;44(6):585–92.

52. van Eps AW, Poulsen L, Belknap JK. The effect of continuous digital hypothermia on lamellar energy metabolism and perfusion during the development of laminitis in the oligofructose model. Abstracts from the 12th International equine colic research Symposium July 18–20, Lexington KY. 2017:38.

53. Belknap JK, Giguere S, Pettigrew A, et al. Lamellar pro-inflammatory cytokine expression patterns in laminitis at the developmental stage and at the onset of lameness: Innate vs. adaptive immune response. Equine Vet J 2007;39(1):42–7.

54. Black SJ, Lunn DP, Yin C, et al. Leukocyte emigration in the early stages of laminitis. Vet Immunol Immunopathol 2006;109(1–2):161–6.

55. Blikslager AT, Yin C, Cochran AM, et al. Cyclooxygenase expression in the early stages of equine laminitis: a cytologic study. J Vet Intern Med 2006;20(5):1191–6.

56. Faleiros RR, Johnson PJ, Nuovo GJ, et al. Laminar leukocyte accumulation in horses with carbohydrate overload-induced laminitis. J Vet Intern Med 2011; 25(1):107–15.
57. Leise BS, Faleiros RR, Watts M, et al. Laminar inflammatory gene expression in the carbohydrate overload model of equine laminitis. Equine Vet J 2011;43(1): 54–61.
58. Burns TA, Westerman T, Nuovo GJ, et al. Role of oxidative tissue injury in the pathophysiology of experimentally induced equine laminitis: a comparison of 2 models. J Vet Intern Med 2011;25(3):540–8.
59. Faleiros RR, Stokes AM, Eades SC, et al. Assessment of apoptosis in epidermal lamellar cells in clinically normal horses and those with laminitis. Am J Vet Res 2004;65(5):578–85.
60. Loftus JP, Johnson PJ, Belknap JK, et al. Leukocyte-derived and endogenous matrix metalloproteinases in the lamellae of horses with naturally acquired and experimentally induced laminitis. Vet Immunol Immunopathol 2009;129(3–4): 221–30.
61. Wang L, Pawlak EA, Johnson PJ, et al. Expression and activity of collagenases in the digital laminae of horses with carbohydrate overload-induced acute laminitis. J Vet Intern Med 2014;28(1):215–22.
62. Bertin FR, Ruffin-Taylor D, Stewart AJ. Insulin dysregulation in horses with systemic inflammatory response syndrome. J Vet Intern Med 2018;32(4):1420–7.
63. Bailey SR, Adair HS, Reinemeyer CR, et al. Plasma concentrations of endotoxin and platelet activation in the developmental stage of oligofructose-induced laminitis. Vet Immunol Immunopathol 2009;129(3–4):167–73.
64. Virgin JE, Goodrich LR, Baxter GM, et al. Incidence of support limb laminitis in horses treated with half limb, full limb or transfixation pin casts: A retrospective study of 113 horses (2000-2009). Equine Vet J Suppl 2011;(40):7–11.
65. Baxter GM, Morrison S. Complications of unilateral weight bearing. Vet Clin North Am Equine Pract 2008;24(3):621–42, ix.
66. Peloso JG, Cohen ND, Walker MA, et al. Case-control study of risk factors for the development of laminitis in the contralateral limb in equidae with unilateral lameness. J Am Vet Med Assoc 1996;209(10):1746–9.
67. Levine DG, Richardson DW. Clinical use of the locking compression plate (LCP) in horses: a retrospective study of 31 cases (2004-2006). Equine Vet J 2007; 39(5):401–6.
68. van Eps A, Collins SN, Pollitt CC. Supporting limb laminitis. Vet Clin North Am Equine Pract 2010;26(2):287–302.
69. Hood DM, Wagner IP, Taylor DD, et al. Voluntary limb-load distribution in horses with acute and chronic laminitis. Am J Vet Res 2001;62(9):1393–8.
70. Thomason JJ, McClinchey HL, Faramarzi B, et al. Mechanical behavior and quantitative morphology of the equine laminar junction. Anat Rec A Discov Mol Cell Evol Biol 2005;283(2):366–79.
71. Thomason JJ, Faramarzi B, Revill A, et al. Quantitative morphology of the equine laminar junction in relation to capsule shape in the forehoof of standardbreds and thoroughbreds. Equine Vet J 2008;40(5):473–80.
72. Faramarzi B. Morphological spectrum of primary epidermal laminae in the forehoof of thoroughbred horses. Equine Vet J 2011;43(6):732–6.
73. Lancaster LS, Bowker RM, Mauer WA. Density and morphologic features of primary epidermal laminae in the feet of three-year-old racing quarter horses. Am J Vet Res 2007;68(1):11–9.
74. Wattle O, Pollitt CC. Lamellar metabolism. Clin Tech Eq Pract 2004;3:22–33.

75. Medina-Torres CE, Pollitt CC, Underwood C, et al. Equine lamellar energy metabolism studied using tissue microdialysis. Vet J 2014;201(3):275–82.

76. Pawlak EA, Geor RJ, Watts MR, et al. Regulation of hypoxia-inducible factor-1alpha and related genes in equine digital lamellae and in cultured keratinocytes. Equine Vet J 2014;46(2):203–9.

77. French KR, Pollitt CC. Equine laminitis: Glucose deprivation and MMP activation induce dermo-epidermal separation in vitro. Equine Vet J 2004;36(3):261–6.

78. Van Kraayenburg FJ. A comparative study of haemodynamics in the equid digit. Theses: The University of Pretoria; 1982.

79. Van Kraayenburg FJ, Fairall N, Littlejohn A. The effect of vertical force on blood flow in the palmar arteries of the horse. In: 1st International Congress on equine exercise physiology, Cambridge. 1983:144-154.

80. Medina-Torres CE, Underwood C, Pollitt CC, et al. The effect of weightbearing and limb load cycling on equine lamellar perfusion and energy metabolism measured using tissue microdialysis. Equine Vet J 2016;48(1):114–9.

81. Wei T, Li WW, Guo TZ, et al. Post-junctional facilitation of substance P signaling in a tibia fracture rat model of complex regional pain syndrome type I. Pain 2009; 144(3):278–86.

82. Jones E, Vinuela-Fernandez I, Eager RA, et al. Neuropathic changes in equine laminitis pain. Pain 2007;132(3):321–31.

83. Collins SN, van Eps AW, Pollitt CC, et al. The lamellar wedge. Vet Clin North Am Equine Pract 2010,26(1):179–95.

84. Ramos JR, Pabijan J, Garcia R, et al. The softening of human bladder cancer cells happens at an early stage of the malignancy process. Beilstein J Nanotechnol 2014;5:447–57.

85. Savagner P. Epithelial-mesenchymal transitions: From cell plasticity to concept elasticity. Curr Top Dev Biol 2015;112:273–300.

86. Lane HE, Burns TA, Hegedus OC, et al. Lamellar events related to insulin-like growth factor-1 receptor signalling in two models relevant to endocrinopathic laminitis. Equine Vet J 2017;49(5):643–54.

87. Wattle O, Ekfalck A, Funkquist B, et al. Behavioural studies in healthy ponies subjected to short-term forced recumbency aiming at an adjunctive treatment in an acute attack of laminitis. Zentralbl Veterinarmed A 1995;42(1):62–8.

88. Moore JN, Vandenplas ML. Is it the systemic inflammatory response syndrome or endotoxemia in horses with colic? Vet Clin North Am Equine Pract 2014;30(2): 337–51, vii-viii.

89. de la Rebiere de Pouyade G, Grulke S, Detilleux J, et al. Evaluation of low-molecular-weight heparin for the prevention of equine laminitis after colic surgery. J Vet Emerg Crit Care (San Antonio) 2009;19(1):113–9.

90. Uberti B, Pressler BM, Alkabes SB, et al. Effect of heparin administration on urine protein excretion during the developmental stage of experimentally induced laminitis in horses. Am J Vet Res 2010;71(12):1462–7.

91. van Eps AW, Leise BS, Watts M, et al. Digital hypothermia inhibits early lamellar inflammatory signalling in the oligofructose laminitis model. Equine Vet J 2012; 44(2):230–7.

92. Durham AE, Frank N, McGowan CM, et al. ECEIM consensus statement on equine metabolic syndrome. J Vet Intern Med 2019;33(2):335–49.

93. Miranda L, Carpentier S, Platek A, et al. AMP-activated protein kinase induces actin cytoskeleton reorganization in epithelial cells. Biochem Biophys Res Commun 2010;396(3):656–61.

94. Zhang L, Li J, Young LH, et al. AMP-activated protein kinase regulates the assembly of epithelial tight junctions. Proc Natl Acad Sci U S A 2006;103(46):17272–7.
95. Kimura N, Tokunaga C, Dalal S, et al. A possible linkage between AMP-activated protein kinase (AMPK) and mammalian target of rapamycin (mTOR) signalling pathway. Genes Cells 2003;8(1):65–79.
96. Burns TA, Watts MR, Weber PS, et al. Laminar inflammatory events in lean and obese ponies subjected to high carbohydrate feeding: Implications for pasture-associated laminitis. Equine Vet J 2015;47(4):489–93.
97. Tomlinson DC, Baxter EW, Loadman PM, et al. FGFR1-induced epithelial to mesenchymal transition through MAPK/PLCgamma/COX-2-mediated mechanisms. PLoS One 2012;7(6):e38972.
98. van Eps AW, Pollitt CC, Underwood C, et al. Continuous digital hypothermia initiated after the onset of lameness prevents lamellar failure in the oligofructose laminitis model. Equine Vet J 2014;46:625–30.

Printed and bound by CPI Group (UK) Ltd, Croydon, CR0 4YY

03/10/2024

01040484-0017